The Power of

Sex

and

How to Wield

It.

By

Samantha Collins

Copyright © 2017 by The Muses' Port Organization, LLC

Written 2017 by Samantha Collins, Published 2017

Jacket designed by Janis Chance and Samantha Collins

ISBN 978-1544020266, 1544020260

First Paperback Edition.

Introduction

The writing of this book have been on my mind for a few years. The reason being is I see so many so called advice books out there about how to get a man, and how to keep him. If you wish. Too many skip the vital parts in building a relationship and go straight to the gusto. Sex. If sex alone could keep a couple together then there wouldn't be so many break ups. It's going to take more than sex to make any relationship work.

And if people knew the true power of sex they wouldn't have it with just anyone and treat it as a recreational sport.

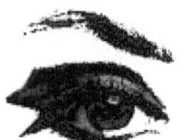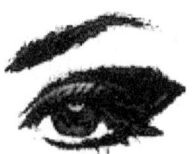

Chapter 1

SEX IS A VERY POWERFUL WEAPON

The Power of Sex is ubiquitously seen every day.
We see it everywhere. From commercials to movies to
books. How often have we purchased something simply
because the model displaying the product was very
attractive? It happens all the time. We buy it without
knowing if the product is useful nor will it work. Yet, in
modern times very few people truly know how to wield
it although we're daily bombard with messages about
love and relationships that has very little for dealing
with real relationships in the real world. In real life, a
situation can not be resolved in thirty minutes to an hour
as in your favorite television show. These storied tactics
only works in fantasy worlds where there's a narrator
controlling the outcome.

This book goes beyond that. It talks about real life
dating, love, marriage, and relationships of all sorts

issues related to human interaction. As everyone knows it's truly a jungle out there and dating and finding love today is much more difficult than in much earlier times. I heard someone say that since sex has become so easy to obtain love has become much harder to find.

But it can be found. One must savvy be willing to take the time and weed out the bad apples and keep the sweet ones. Don't let desperation and despair keep you from continuing to search for the one who is good for you and to you.

The media and commercial uses the power of sex everyday. Why? Because sex sells. Simple as that! They display their products as being sexy because everyone wants to be sexy. Everyone wants the opposite gender to find them attractive. It's a basic human need. This need exists in the animal kingdom as well.

"The Power of Sex and How to Wield it" is based upon years of experience in dealing with the opposite gender and the human race in general. As to what I have known to work and what doesn't. It is not a sex manual. There are many sex manuals out there. Everyone already knows the rope in getting a person in bed. There isn't of anything which can be added to that. But since sex has become more plenteously and easier to attain. The art of finding love, enjoying an embraceable romance, taking the time to conduct a real courtship and creating a lasting relationship is dying and on life support.

It's isn't a manual showing one how to use sex to lead to love and a lasting relationship. Because rarely does that happens. Although, sex is the real reason for the male's introducing himself but it must develop beyond the initial motivation to flourish.

I heard a gasp. Let's be frank here ladies. Even those of you who are married and have been married for years I'm sorry to burst your illusion. But the first time your husband spoke to you or asked you out. It was sex he had on the brain as his reason for asking you out on a date. It eventually blossomed into something deeper as to why he asked you to be his wife. If sex was not on his brain the wedding night wouldn't be the highlight of the day he married you. Truth be told. I know he isn't going to tell it but he doesn't rightly remember what the minister or justice asked him during the ceremony nor does he truly remember what either of you said in your vows. All the decorations of the wedding and wedding reception are endured for your sake. Because he loves you and wanted to make you happy while in reality, as far as he's concerned; things could go from the altar to the bedroom. Skip all else in between. He may not remember the color of your garter but he remembers every detail of the wedding night and the honeymoon. Why? Because these two are about the primary reason he married you.

Chapter 2

WHAT IS EXACTLY IS SEX AND WHY IS IT SO IMPORTANT??

We hear about it all day long. Every day of the week.

It's the subjected whisper about in pillow talk. Lewd jokes are made about it. Empires have risen and fallen upon it. Laws are made to govern it. Wars have been fought over it. Many has been killed in the name of it. The sale of it is the world's oldest profession.

So why is it so important to us? Or to any living creature? First of all, it's how our species continues from one generation to the next. It's how the human race attain immortality. Our ancestors who lived 12 million years ago are still alive today through us. Their traits, habits, chromosomes and elements of their bodies are still alive in us.

Secondly, sex is actual a natural process and need. Most people heed the need to procreate. It's the way we procreate the next generation. It's how we become immortal through our offsprings and those of our siblings. The first and second reason if you note are interchangeable. But lucky for us humans the need isn't a destructive one. It isn't the same as with animals. We can control or urges without violence and mayhem. Well, most of us can and we have law to govern those who can not. Or at least say they can not.

It satisfies an emotional need that exist within all humans. All humans have a desire to be loved. Sex is one of the ways we express that desire and fulfill the need for love in another human being.

You may have asked if it's a need, then why all the stigmatization of it? Why all the secrecy and salacious comments about it when sex is as much a natural biological function such as eating, sleeping and all mammals participates? So why is it such a mystery when it's something natural? Why is it governed by the social norms of society?

First of all, some laws need to be in place to govern those who choose not to conform to the normalcy of relationships and not resort to violence. Normalcy doesn't mean anything goes because an individual feels it's normal. For example, some may feel normal to rape and sexually abuse others. That doesn't fall under the guideline of normalcy. Consequently, rape is so often presented as being about sex. While in reality, rape is rarely about sex. It's all about wielding power and sadly it is one of the ultimate ways sex is used as a weapon. The act itself is about power, control, humiliation and often times resulting in death.

To answers the questions above I believe that in the Western world and many other parts of the world people have not been taught it is a normal part of being human. There's nothing lewd or salacious about it. No one tries to humiliate anyone for eating or breathing. I mean sane people. I'm leaving the insane out the context. I believe these disturbing definitions come into play when other sought ways to use it was a weapon to control and manipulate others.

I firmly believe the reason the patriarch system came into existence is that the females for thousands of years had the upper hand in society. The reason being is that the female of all species has the upper hand in this agenda is our ability to give birth. But they fail to realized that without this ability of the females... no amount of laws would be necessary for there would be no one to govern.

But somewhere along the line things switched places and we are now living in a patriarchal society where the male is supposed to have the upper hand. This belief system has causes a severe contrast to reality and illusion. That man can not exist alone as many of the patriarchal teaching would have men to believe he can.

If we listen to the patriarch system every god in the world hates women and is out to punish them. Punish them for what? According to the patriarch system none of the powerful celestial beings are women. I sat and thought about that one day and that doesn't sound right. If none are women....then is Nirvana, Heaven or where ever your religious final destination maybe___are they places filled with nothing but men walking around? I remember reading a scripture speaking of *"Those who have defiled themselves with women."* From what I gathered it was saying women are some filthy sub-creatures that lying with them, loving one of them will make one unfit for eternal bliss.

I have found so many versions of this misogynistic teaching that makes no logical sense whatsoever. For example, the seventy virgins' scenario...why would you want to spend eternity with 70 people you don't know? Where will they come from? How do you know they will like you? Will they be divinely programed to love you? To me that doesn't sound very appealing. As far as you know the seventy virgins could be a bunch of guys. The religious text didn't specify gender.

The reason I researched different world religions when gathering material for this book is that religion plays a vital role in the development and conduct of all social and cultural norms and can constructive or destructive. I believes that anything that teaches discrimination, oppression, depraved ideas of anyone regardless of any gender or sexual orientation is not one of love. In love, there's no place for oppression nor discrimination.

Chapter 3

KNOWLEDGE IS POWER

Keeping one ignorant of their power makes it far easier to control them and make them into whatever you wish them to be. It's sad, even today so many women knows so little about their body and how it function. Why? Because they have been taught from infancy that their vaginas are something separate from themselves. It's bad. It's filthy. It's a problematic organ that need not to exist.

Men do not feel the same way about their penis. Most are very proud of it. They have been taught to be proud of it. Proud of being male. For it is cursed to be female and thanks to whatever god who made them saw fit to make them male.

From the way things are presented, from the way it is told that females are the reason the world is in such shambles. That Eve sinned in Eden. I have a problem with this one because it is hard to get your husband to take out the trash so how was she so crafty that she persuaded her husband to something no other woman had been able to do. Eat something he didn't want to eat. Her daughters have been trying ever since to get men to do something they don't want to do. Has it worked? No. So, she need to return and show us all how she did it?

The second problem I have with this is that I've seen no proof of. It's mostly males who declare wars, kill, and main each other. Not women. We bitch at each other a lot but rarely does we kill each other.

My theory of how ancient societies changed from matriarchal to patriarchal is some catastrophic event took place severely disrupting the order of things. Forcing human to rely on physical strength for survival at the time of the great cultural change of systems of the human race from a matriarchal to a patriarchal rule. This apparently happened approximately ten thousand years ago for Picts left behind prior to the last ice age shows that there were far more emphases were placed on goddesses not gods. So what happened? Again, my theory is some natural event occurred that threaten the existence of the human race in some areas and the male being the strongest of the gender took over and led the way. And seeing we needed them to survive they got the big head and decided this is how it was going to be from this day forth. After scrutinizing many records the only event I came across that affected the entire globe was the last Ice Age, itself.

I read one theory stating this change took place about the time man figured out his role in reproduction. I don't buy that one. I believe man have always known his role in reproduction. As fascinated as most men are with their penis, I didn't believe they just figured out what it was for in the last ten to eight thousand years. There're are ancient cities where there're penis shaped sculptures all over. These monuments were built signifying the potent of the city. They wore penis-shaped pendants around their neck and hung them sons' necks. So no, ancient man knew its' purpose was more than to urinate.

Whatever happened in the last ten to eight thousand years put women in a binder. It may make men suffer but the patriarch rule oppresses women and distort how women see themselves. Although, no society can reach its fullest potential nor greatest height oppressing one half of it's citizens. If the Picts of old taught us anything, it's not to repeat what caused the ancient civilizations to fail. We don't know exactly what happened but whatever happened, didn't fall in favor of the female gender.

Chapter 4
LOVE THY SELF

The first and foremost lesson to be learned in learning to wield the power of sex is learning to love yourself. If you can not see yourself as lovable then others can not and will not see you as loveable either. You must love who you see in the mirror every morning before you can attempt to love someone else. Self love can serve as a guideline of your expectations and acceptances in a relationship. Loving oneself has nothing to do with being narcissistic nor conceited. Nor does it have anything to do with being arrogance or being puffed up with so much pride it's rumbling somewhere in that warped mind of yours you're better than everyone else and others should bow at your feet.

What loving yourself means is knowing and asserting your worth and letting no one take it from you. This is important because too often people do not feel their worth and get involved with others who can see they do not know their worth and unfortunately there are unscrupulous individuals who will take advantage of this aspect.

Lack of self love drives too many women to accept men into their lives who really couldn't be there. Lack of self love accounts for too many women handing over their most precious possession, their body, along with control and power to a man who abuses it. Lack of self love cause too many women to remain with men who are physical abusive for whatever reason. Lack of self love equals lack of confident.

Self love builds confidence and self-confidence is a very important aspect in achieving your goals of finding whomever is meant for you. No, I don't as if is written in the stars' kind of '*meant for you*'. I mean find whomever is compatible with you. Whomever is willing to love you for who you are and as you deserve to be loved.

S

One of the hottest and depressing trends nowadays on the relationship circuit is being a man's side chick. Why on earth would any woman settle for being someone's else leftovers? I interviewed a few involved in this sort of relationship and some say they do not wish to be in a committed relationship. Don't worry, it will never happen. But in reality, the truth is lack of self love is reason why. Why would you want to sleep with someone who will never take you to meet his family or spend the holidays with you?

Sadly too many women enter these relationships and accept the second-handed loving believing all the best guys are already taken. That is not true, it maybe the case in your community but there are hundreds of men willing to talk to you and treat you how your married or committed boyfriend can not and will not treat you. He's never going to leave his wife or girlfriend no matter what he says or how sweet it sounds.

But I found in each of these women a common thread and that was lack of self-esteem. Some have been hurt so badly so many times they're afraid to get involved in a committed relationship because of all the heart and mind games played today. The married or committed guy is safe. At least they think so until they slip up and find themselves in love with him and he refuses to leave the supposedly love of his life.

Too often people enters relationships to fix this aspect

of their life. And when they don't get it in a relationship they blame the other person for not fixing it. Not loving them enough. First of all, they entered the relationship for all the wrong reasons. They entered with the feeling they needed to see themselves through the eyes of someone who loves them. There was nothing wrong with this. Infants learn to feel loved through how those around them sees them and treat them. Even pets learn they are loved in pretty much the same manner. All humans need love and to see themselves through the eyes of others to be human and feel loved. It's one of the greatest gift one human can give another but don't become bitter, despair and withdraw from life if you do not get it. Two broken people can not fix each other. Each must fix themselves.

Some people are fortune enough to find someone who loves them eventhus they don't love themselves. But it doesn't happen as often as Hollywood would have to believe it does. That is very rare as to why I say *'love yourself if no one else loves you'*.

Love yourself and others will see that they too will have to love you if they wish to be in your company. This is one agenda where you set the rules and can exclude anyone who refuses to follow them. True, you can't force anyone to love you but you don't have to tolerate anyone who don't.

Chapter 5

IF YOU THINK YOU'RE SEXY OTHERS WILL TOO.

Now, I'm getting to the second most important piece advice. If you think you are sexy others will too. Being sexy starts in the mind. In how we see ourselves. Most of us aren't one of those people who are naturally sexy without trying to be sexy. I met such a woman who was sexy as they come from the way she moved to the way she walked but I noticed all of it came naturally and very effortless for her. Well, this isn't most of us. As for most of us we must work at it by developing life long healthy habits and attitudes.

S

However, being sexy is mostly a state of mind moreso than physical appearance as to why I talked so much about social and mental conditionals and cultural and psychological assaults. The most beautiful woman in the world may get a lot of attention but if beauty is her only asset she will eventually lost it. But if she knows she beautiful and knows she sexy then there's no stopping her. Unfortunately, we live in a world where beauty is a valuable asset. But much more is needed to make a serious impression or one that won't come across as shallow and without depths.

S

Psychological and cultural assault undermines the self esteem of far too many women and girls. Depriving them of this very important aspect of being feminine. Being sexy doesn't always means sexual as it is so popular taught. Being sexy doesn't have to always mean sexual active or even attempting to allure a partner although that's the most common definition. Being sexy can simply mean feeling good about oneself. Feeling proud in who you are. Comfortable with being a woman or being feminine.

There appears to be no room in most societies for a woman to simply be who she is in her own space of feminine vice in simply being a woman and not be seen as sexual. Even the very word *"woman"* conjure images of sex. While that is very narrow minded definition it had been the standard for thousands of years.

To defeat this cultural deprivation that starts around the age 10-12 requires being somewhat of a bitch. No, I'm not suggesting that 10-12 year old girls turn into bitches. I'm speaking to their mothers or other females guardians responsible for them. This is approximately the age social begun to try and to force them to conform to its idea of being female. Depriving them of the freedom to be themselves and letting them chose their own idea of femininity. This is approximately the age they start being seriously instructed what's expected of them. Meaning you must look and behave in a ladylike manner to be accepted. There's nothing wrong with acting like a lady, but let the girl decides if that's the mode that's right for her. Not society decides it. She'll have many years to grow into the world's idea of femininity. But sadly, too many parents push their daughters into this mode during their early teen years without considering whether or not she wants to be the sexy girl in junior high or high school.

Chapter 6

YOU CAN'T KEEP SOMEONE WHO DOESN'T WANT TO BE KEPT.

Now, I'm getting to another piece of advice. You can't keep anyone who doesn't want to be kept by you or be with you. I'm mentioning this because there has been an increase in relationships suicides of both male and females in the past twenty years. If you have jump through flaming hoops to keep him or her happy. You are better off without them. Yes, any successful relationship requires work but shouldn't feel like you're out digging an old-fashioned well.

Once I was talking to a man who had been married for over thirty years who hadn't exactly been faithful to his wife but after thirty years she walked away. After her departure; he became suicidal. I asked him did over the years she learn of his numerous affairs? He admitted she did. Then I asked him why are you attempting to kill yourself when it was you who killed your own marriage? He didn't have an answer my question. I'm not saying this is the case with every single break up but usually there's something sending signals as vigilance as fireworks signaling the end is approaching.

I won't deny break-ups and divorces are very painful. But no one is worth giving your life for. Cry, scream, pitch a tantrum if you must to relieve yourself of the pain. But always remember, you lived before you met them therefore you can live on after they are gone. Do anything but off yourself. I wish whomever reads this, who is considering this act just stop and please think.

"Were the significant already exhibiting signals they wanted out and I ignored them? Did I do something such as take them for granted, cheat on them or abuse to force their action. Or were if they were even a good companion?"

Sometimes none of the above applies. Their reason for being with you may no longer seem lucrative to them. It doesn't mean because it ended it wasn't a good relationship while it lasted. It means that many factors may have contributed to the break up. Sometimes people simply grow apart even they have the best of intentions to stay together.

But as Mandy Hale said,, "Sometimes it takes a heartbreak to shake us awake and help us see we are worth so much more than we're settling for."

Chapter 7

A LOT OF THE ADVICE I'VE SEEN NOWADAYS DEMANDS TOO MUCH OF THE WOMAN AND

NOT ENOUGH OF THE MAN.

Once in between marriages, while at the airport on my way to London to see a boyfriend I hadn't seen in three months I picked up one of these self-help books at the airport. I finished it before landing at Heathrow but I told myself, "there's no way in hell am I following the advice of that book." My boyfriend would think I was nuts or something terrible happened to me if I followed the advice in this book.

The advice was after I've weary towed, lugged heavy luggage of out an apartment into a cab, lugged them to the airport, checked them in and have flown all the way across the vast Atlantic Ocean and repeated the same procedures as at the JFK airport that I perform sexual aerobatic moves in bed while kissing his ass the moment I dropped my suitcases at his flat. I'm serious, that was the equivalence of what they were saying. That I was wrong for making him pay for the cab fares, tickets, dinner, shopping expedition and again taking me to dinner my entire time there and on a tour of London before sleeping with him. According to this article I was doing it all backward and I was gold-digger. Wow! I didn't know that! I didn't know I was supposed to have rubbed his feet and shoulders. Be willing to dine on fish and chips under London Bridge if he wanted to. Make him feel good and then asked for nothing. Not even a plane ticket back the USA. Not that I had to ask for these things. But according to the article I just read our get-together was supposed to be all about him. I was only there four days because I had to return to work after the holidays. I wanted to see London so he sent for me. I thought he was doing what a boyfriend supposed to do but the relationship article said I had it all wrong.

Let me start by telling you who I'm and what under authority I'm writing from. First of all, I'm not wealthy or a celebrity, I'm not a sex talk show host. I'm not sex therapist, not I'm not a sugar baby, I'm not famous but I have been proposed to more times than Elizabeth Taylor and have accepted two of them. And have over ten diamond rings to prove it. No, none of the men asked for the rings back and yes, they were all real diamonds. I have been all over the world and never once paid for a flight ticket. A few times I have paid for the cab fare. I have been given gifts ranging from cars to designer handbags to clothing, furniture to houses, additional to the furs and jewelry. Never once did I chase the man or do any of these things the popular magazine suggested. Never once did I go out and find the apartment or house, the man I was with did it every time. I merely moved in. And no, I didn't have to act like a bitch to get any of these things. So, with all that said. I think I'm qualified to give advice on the subject. I must be doing something right.

I don't consider myself the most beautiful woman in the world but I know how to make a man think that I'm.

So far from what I have read in the plethoras of sex-relationship books that gives advice....most of it is something I've never used. Sex only keep his attention for a while. You can't sex a man into loving you. All the sex tricks in the world will eventually wear off him if you have nothing else to offer. Because all women have a pussy and yours isn't as special as you believe and men aren't peculiar about whose pussy they are in just so long the woman has one. Sure, they lie to us and say they wouldn't sleep with the such and such woman we think we are superior to and will turns right around and crawl in her bed.

Trying to gain affection through sex only gains you a broken heart and nothing more and in some cases. But can also it gains you children you can not afford with a father who doesn't want them nor you. It's not worth the drama.

The advice I have read so popular today for women. A man must have written it or a woman who was born into wealth where her reputation can easily be repaired by mother or father's money. But for the average women those suggesting are dating and finding a suitable mate suicide.

I've read the same advice over and over so no one can say it came strictly from their articles or book for it's all over the place. They are telling women to take the lead in sexual matters. But I'm wondering does they realize with a man...a relationship has to have reached a certain stage before this can be effective?? They tell women to not be afraid to be rule in the situation. To be the first to initiate sexual contact. To get the man follow your lead sexually. Many men find this arousing and enjoy sex more with women who display sexual confidence. Blah, blah, blah.

This rarely works if you are trying to allure him to you to start a serious relationship. Sure, any guy will follow you to a bedroom or behind a building or anywhere to have sex with you. But being overly dominate can kill their desire for you once he's finished.

I'm not suggesting anyone to be a wallflower, I'm

suggesting letting him come to you. Send him signals if you're interested. Most men are intelligent enough to catch the hint. The eyes can speak volumes across a room or streets. One woman said she tried this and the man of her interested turned up his nose and looked disgust and mortified at her and walked away. Well, sometimes it can be that way especially in areas where the men are catered to as if they emperors or perhaps he was gay. Whatever the reason he did it I told her don't let one guy determine nor defer you.

  These are the kind of things you do once you are in a firm, solid relationship. Sure, pull out the sexy lingerie and such, set the table for romance to let him know what's on your mind. It doesn't take acting out to let him know. Most guys assume that's what's you want from your simply asking them to help you change the sheets when no, you really want him on the other side tucking the sheet in so you won't have to keep walking round the bed to do it. But they assume sex is your *real* reason for inviting him into the bedroom at 10:00 on a Sunday morning.

Where are these men who needs all this arousal and encouragement? I have no idea. I've never met one. Perhaps they are in a nursing home on life support without access to Viagra. That much be it as to why I haven't seen one yet.

Men are hunters and chasers by natural. I say it's for the survival of our species. So in the beginning let him think he's doing the pursuing even if he isn't.

S

Another piece of new trendy advice I found but sorely disagree with; buying him gifts. A card or scarf will be sufficient enough until the relationship is cemented. Giving a guy expensive gifts and flowers he is going to run. Well, most men who are relationship material will run. This practice attracts users who will take the gifts and still leave.

I say this is because a man will let you know how he

feels about you by what he is willing to do for you. Men express their affection by actions. They feel it's their duty to bring and buy you things. They feel that in you doing so, you are taking the manly role from them and they don't like that. Yes, yes, I know that sound old fashioned but it's the truth. Young women, (meaning the millennium crowd) there's nothing wrong with a young man showing his affection by bringing you gifts or flowers. Remember...wherever a man is laying is his wallet is where his heart will soon follow. His monetary investments show where his heart is. I know this is so violently denied today. But it still holds true regardless of what the popular trends says. If he shows up empty handed then his heart is empty of any real, lasting intimate emotions for you. Yes, I'm aware there are players who comes bearing gift. But they are usually something non-personal and usually very cheap. I'm not talking about a millionaire who spending a couple thousand means nothing to him. I'm talking about the average guy.

There's something coded into them that makes them wants to bring you things. Long ago they used to bring food they harvested or hunted down and killed to the woman of their interest. Just as there's nothing wrong with allowing them to hold a door open for you, it does nothing to your independence as a modern woman. It doesn't mean a damn thing. It's simply common courtesy not to let the door fall in someone's face.

Chapter 8

EXPOSED TO TOO MUCH SEX TO SOON.

When doing research for this book I came across some sexual scenes online that was traumatizing to me. So, I can't imagine how desensitizing this must be to a preteen.

No boy eight or nine years old needs to be watching a woman push a baby out her vagina. Simple as that. This is far too much too soon. He'll have plenty of time for that once he's help delivering his own children. The women who post such pictures I wish I could find them all and shake them until their teeth rattles. Shake some sense into them. They aren't doing womanhood a favor. Childbirth is a private event not a sporting spectacular for the entire world to see. I saw one video where this crazy woman had her sons in the birthing room with her. It would have been ok if the children had been daughters of at least 10 to 12 but 8 and 9 year old sons? Those boys are going to grow into young men who are never going to be able to talk to and relate to women without seeing a vagina pushing a baby out. What in the hell is wrong with people like that?

I'm not a prude but I do believe there are certain boundaries you do not cross and that is one of them.

S

Another popular trend that was popular even when I was junior high back in the 90's. Girls performing oral sex on a regular basis on 'all the boys they loved' to prevent pregnancy. The more she's willing to perform it the more popular she becomes until everyone has had their spritz and then drop her like a hot frying pan. I wondered then as I wonders now...who told these girls that this was a way to get and hold on to a boy? And where are their parents or guardians? Sure, my parents worked but I better not have had a boy in their house while they were at work. I had to come straight home from school and better stay there until my parents came home from work.

S

Don't get me started on those whom I call the internet "Flashers." You find them everywhere. They will show you their penis, vagina or anus with no reservation. They are everywhere you don't want them to be. I think too many young people are being exposed to this and it has desensitized them in respecting the fact that sex is something more than a physical encounter. Most are not mature enough to handle to emotional impact of it. Most has never known what it's like to have a crush on somebody. Most have never known what is like to date someone wasn't immediately courting the aspect of having sex with them. They know nothing about puppy love or innocent love. It's not their fault we adults didn't work harder to protect them from the overexposure to the freak and fetish shows. It's our fault. Sure, it is hard to supervisor their every move but if we can attend to other adults' business, we can get off our asses and see what's going on with our youth.

My heart goes out to the teenage girls who doesn't know that video of her shaking her ass to anyone who wants to look have severely damaged her chances in becoming anyone's wife or serious love interest. Men and boys start to review her as good enough to striptease but not good enough to be his wife or take home to their family.

Some argues that strip club women do it all the time so what's the big deal. She's getting paid and is most likely an adult and you are not. I even had one to argue it was common in some parts of the world to nude dance or twerp. Maybe but she didn't live in that part of the world and the societies where it's a common ceremonial dance, it isn't just a sexual dance. It's a fertility dance.

S

It's sad so many teenager girls think that having slept

with more guys than her age is alright and even viewed as status symbol among her peers. They're too young to realize it has nothing to do with love and all that is fun is not a game. I know they are really seeking love, attention and affection, and learned at an early age that sex gets them a short span of attention and false display of affection for a while. But men talk and her name has been passed on as being a nothing more than a vagina in case anyone nearby is looking for free sex. The ones sleeping with her they don't even care enough to try to defer other males by saying she had a venereal disease. Which I know would be wrong to say but they don't care enough to say anything.

To make it all worst most of her sexual partners aren't teenage boys. Most are fully grown men. Oftentimes with daughters of their own her age. And yes, many of these lovers are married men. The girls consider proudly themselves *the side chick'*. I would like to point out that his epidemic has no social-economic barriers before any one blatantly dismiss it as merely a ghetto or poor girl thing.

All of this is a result of too much exposure to sex too early in life with no real parental supervision. Children aren't mentally equipped to handle this gross overload of pure sexuality coming at them from all directions. From everything from the internet to television. Sex is being blaring at them on a daily basis. It seriously affects how they learn to relate to the opposite gender.

S

What I found is that it especially effected the young men view of women. Some has been so desensitized toward vaginal sex that it longer holds any fascination for them. Several told me something I would've never guessed. They've tried homosexuality too but they don't consider themselves gay all because women have lost their appear to them. They said they don't have to ask a woman or girl for sex. That oftentimes it is she who comes to him not he goes to her. She gives it to him without asking and have no expectations in return.

All the men I surveyed were under 25 years old. (18-24 year olds. At leas that's what they said.) I was like *"Wow, you all really do have a very low opinion of women!"*

I grumbled as I put together the information to write this book thinking, "Thanks to you so-called dating and sex advice specialists and your weird ass advice and pointers and everyone throwing sex around like confetti in a parade; now we have an entire generation of young people who are completely desensitized to a loving sexual relationship and thinks sex is as recreational as playing a video game. All you did was taught the girls how to give away the only real power a woman has in this world and the boys not to appreciate, respect, nor cherish it."

Chapter 9

WHAT MEN FIND THE MOST ATTRACTIVE ABOUT A WOMAN?

The single biggest attractive trait most men find in a

woman is how she carries herself. To most men, it's your self confident that they find is the sexiest thing about a woman. Her, being comfortable in her own skin. It doesn't matter how beautiful you are, what color your skin or eyes maybe. Nor how intelligent you are or how well you can speak. He will never find out any of these things if you are wallowing in low self esteem.

Guys can spot low esteem a mile away and runs like hell from it. Beware there are predators out there who seeks out women with low self-esteem to victimize and use for his pleasure until he grows weary of her. There are entire sex industries built upon the backs of women with low self-esteem. It's far more common than most people care to know.

Chapter 10

BEING A BITCH IS EXACTLY WHAT IT SOUNDS LIKE. BEING A BITCH!

Being modest isn't the same as having low esteem or allowing others to walk all over you. Being modest is knowing when to assert oneself, speak up, and make demands and knowing when to remain silence. Being modest comes in handy at times just as being a first class bitch comes in handy at times. But being one or the other 24/7 is a sure relationship killers.

Being modest at all times when one should be a first class bitch is only going to gain you the label of being a doormat or a pushover and taken for granted.

Being a bitch 24/7 is only going to attract men with low self-esteem or men who likes to be dominated. The Alpha males whom all women drool over are usually not attracted to bitchy women. Just as a woman who has a healthy opinion of herself isn't going to tolerate a guy who acts like a bastard 24/7, then a well adjusted man isn't going to tolerate a 24/7 bitch. He may chase you. He may even marry you but there will come one day he is going to get feed up with your bitchiness and walk away.

Too many women feel that being an ultra bitch is the only way to get what you need in life. They're so wrong. All it get you is lots of enemies. Being a bitch isn't the same as being assertive or telling someone what you want or need. Nor is it standing up for yourself. Being a bitch is exactly what it sounds like and is. Being a bitch. There's no nice way to say this. Which is why I always fairly warns people, please don't be a bitch to me because I'll reciprocate it and I can do it much better than you.

Being modest or being a lady doesn't mean being mousy, a shrinking violet, nor a pushover. Being modest means respecting yourself and demanding respect in return and cutting loose anyone who refuses to respect you. Unfortunately, occasionally you have to let the bitch side of you come out to get your point across. Yes, there will be times in life when being a bitch is a must. But don't make it a lifestyle.

Chapter 11

RESPECT-WHAT DOES IT MEANS TO YOU?

I place a lot of emphasis on respect because we as a society have lost our way with all aspects of it. You can not get love out of a society of rude and disrespectful people. That just isn't going to happen. We've accepted rudeness as being normal or even cool and sophisticated and then wonders why love is so hard to find? It doesn't take a genius to figure out where's the love has gone? It went out the window with respect.

Disrespect has become so common-place and that even certain derogatory words has become a term of endearments. It has become a term of endearment to call a woman a bitch. Words like whore, slut, shank, cunt are now every day and common terms used when referring to women that even a lot of women no longer find them offensive. The recent elections have proven just how little women have come to care about respect being shown for them.

Words like whore, slut, shank, cunt, bitch, nasty, pig,

cow, whale, split tail, pussy are designed to inflict pain, injury, and to insults. They are not terms of endearment. When you allow someone to call you such names do not be surprised when his fist or palm meet your face. Just remember that **disrespect** is always the forerunner of domestic violence.

When women accept this behavior as normal and funny they do not realize they are giving away their power to demand respect. If a man calls you a degrading word he **will** hit you. The two goes hand in hand. So I hope no one is thinking it is something cute or funny when a man says these things. Or believe because of whatever reason unknown to the rest of the universe he will not harm you or he didn't mean it when he said those hateful words. Yes, he did. He meant them or he wouldn't have said them.

Chapter 12

KNOW WHO YOU ARE SLEEPING WITH.

Recently while on a subway coming into New York

City from Connecticut, I'd about a 45 minutes' commute which I usually spent reading but a chatting group sat near me and disturbed my reading solstice. I overheard this group of young people under twenty five speaking and using a lot of SMH, LOL, IMHO. I had nothing against abbreviations when texting but I think they could stay in the text messages. Anyway, I heard them mentioned something called **trcouple or qaudcouple**?

Curiosity got the better of me so I asked what was that? Yes, I'm one of those older people who don't care if you frown and sigh. For I can do it much better. One girl explained to me it's when three or more people are in a relationship.

"Oh, like the 1960's and 70's swinging?" I asked. "Or the hippie communities?"

The girl closest to me turned from her friends and sighed again. I returned it for she was getting on my damn nerves too. All three of them. Two girls and one guy. The situation was one of the girls had stepped out on the group and was dating someone else and the other three felt she was being unfaithful to the union. The young man among the three girl also had male lover who didn't live with the group. Ok, to make a long story short she explained it wasn't like the 1960's and 70's. I asked what was the difference? The guy was getting the best deal back then just this young man is getting the best deal now. So how was him sleeping with all three of you and his boyfriend beneficial to you three young ladies?

The second girl explained they had a real relationship. Unlike the hippie's communal and swingers of the past. And the reason the absent girl was wrong is that they knew nothing about her new lover but they knew about his boyfriend. That people must be careful in the day of AIDS as to who they sleep with.

I agreed that people must be very careful as to who they have sex with nowadays. But I also told her so did the communal groups of the Flower Power Era believe they had a real relationship and were sleeping with everyone as a community but we all see how that turned out so what make you four believe this is going to work better than a monogamous relationship?

They gave me some lame of explanation about how mankind wasn't meant to be a monogamous. To be with only one person their entire life time. That during one's youth is when you discover yourself and find out what you want in life.

I debated I didn't deny your youth was when you experienced with life but there was still limits. Just because you wish to experience doesn't mean things won't have dire consequences down the road. And no one knows for sure what the young man's other partner is doing if he doesn't live with the four of you.

The young man accused me of being homophobia. I told him I am not but you don't know what someone is doing you don't live with and you need to protect your-self so you can protect your lady friends. And why is this always the first accusation when speaking to a gay couple is beyond my comprehension. Being gay doesn't make you immune to any of the ills a heterosexual couple encounters. It's no magical relationship pill.

I was speaking to the young women about protecting themselves because this is not the 1960's and 70's. Today's venereal diseases kill.

They argued that no one knows for sure where their partner(s) have been or who they have slept with. That is very true which is why I advises women to always, duly protect themselves. Do not let the prospect of find love guide you to give away the power to protect your own life.

From what they explained to me it's nothing but a modern hippie communal revised. And very few of those couples from those communes got together for good and if so very few are still together.

Some associate advising women not to freely give

away sex as saying that you in the Puritanical Age and that women could still be stigmatize and denounced for having pre-marital sex. When that is not the case at all. Like it or not, women gave away a lot of power during the Sexual Revolution. I see it as their going about it the wrong way. Men have always wanted to have as much sex with as many women has he should possible rise to the occasion to screw. That's why the rich ones in many nations used to have harems. That's nothing new. But the courtesan, harem, or mistresses of long ago had some power as long as he gave it to her. While on the other hand, the movement of the Sixties and Seventies gave the women nothing out of the relationship but children with no stable homes. No, I'm not a conservative if that is what anyone is wondering.

I've always viewed these women as casualties of the Sexual Revolution although, much was accomplished and benefited the generations of women who followed behind them. And I thank them for making the way for my generation to enjoy the freedom we do. But in the progress they lost much of the power women previously had. They threw away the ability to make strongly men desire women by making sex readily available to men. Anything that comes too easily is rarely appreciated.

Chapter 13

POWDER AND PAINT MAKE YOU WHAT YOU AIN'T.

Have you ever been to a high end party or formal attire gala and noticed there are always a few women all the men crowd around or turn to look at the moment she walks in? What's one thing all these women have in common besides self confidence? The answer is: "Well applied make-up." They all have learned the art of skillfully applying make up to enhance their best features.

Let's be frank very few of us have the skin without blemish and the naturally smoky eyes and the pouty heart shaped mouth that men love to watch move when you are talking.

I know nowadays it's said that wearing make up is being dishonest. The irony in this statement about being open and honest....is how is facial make up and hair extensions dishonest but breast and butt implants aren't according the gospel of men who don't know what in the hell they are talking about? I see it as they aren't interested in your face, hair, nor nails as to why they disagree with enhancing them.

I assume the ancient Geisha must have said, "I don't give a fuck. He's being dishonest too so we will be dishonest together." Even the natural look make up isn't for everyone and is harder to accomplish than most women realize.

One of the powerful features on any woman are her lips. That's what he's watching when talking to you before his eyes travel down the length of your body. A well suited coat of lipstick can make or break your allure. Your lips can be your greatest weapon if made up attractively. There isn't a woman whom lipstick doesn't compliment.

When I say make-up, I don't mean put on so much make-up that you look like a Japanese kabbuki actor. Although, I think the make-up of a kabbuki dancer is beautiful. I don't think it meant to be worn off-stage. And nor do you have to dress like a Cochina Doll. I mean learn to apply it for the right occasion. Light applications of make-up for the day and heavier and more vibrant make-up for the night. For the love of all womankind...throw away those pastel teeny boppers' colors. Those pastel colors make every grown woman look washed out. They are fine for those under 18 but once you're an adult ditch the teen colors. But for a mature woman to still wear the colors she wore as teenager says she hasn't moved beyond her teen years and if I can see that, so can men. They watch women far more intensely than me.

S

I know in a perfect world not ruled by men these things wouldn't matter. But that's a world yet to come. However, there's no way you are going to attract an upward mobility man without showing him your best face, when you get him is the time to show him your natural face. He'll have plenty of time to see it. He'll after your first rendezvous. By then he'll have fallen in love with you and your <u>every</u> face is beautiful in his eyes. I see too many women shows up at formal parties wearing their bare face, and bare legs. No leg covering such as silk stockings, without proper underwear for that particular style of dress, no jewelry and expect to walk off with a millionaire at the end of the evening. Sure, he may walk off into the evening with you for a one-night stand if you present yourself so half-assed. But if you don't take yourself seriously, then neither will he.

No one is so beautiful they don't need help nor improvements. What's the point in wearing a five thousand dollar dress if you aren't going to glamor **yourself** up to match the dress?

I'm going to use an allegory here: All women loves beautiful, well-designed handbags. Now, if your favorite designer put together a bag of an undyed rawhide bag with no silk lining, no decoration, no pockets, nor pouches, it looks like something he or she threw together at the last minute....would you pay $1,200 for it? No, you wouldn't so why could a man invest his time and money in you if you walk around looking like a rawhide handbag? Or if your favorite cereal company just poured the cereal in a plain cardboard box and scribbled their name on it with crayon.... would you buy it and eat it? No, you wouldn't. That would be an insult to you.

Don't follow every fad that comes along. Every fad doesn't compliment every body type. Experiment with styles and fashions and learn what looks best on you and update it as time progress. Don't get stuck in a fashion rut. The classics are always a great buy for they can be easily be updated with something as simple as a new scarf or necklace.

I know you all have heard some men decry the usage

of make-up and jewelry to beautify yourself. Saying that's dishonesty. While the truth it is, it had nothing to do with honesty. It has all to do with money. That's a red flag in what a relationship with him is going to be like. It's warning signal. I hate to say it but it is. He's telling you as plain as it gets; do not expect me to shower you with attention or gifts because it is going to be all about me. He's saying as clearly as it gets he prefers a low maintenance woman who will cook, clean, not question him, have sex whenever he wants it, make no demands. So, it's not the make-up at all that he dislikes. It's what the make up symbolizes which is a challenge to him. It symbolizes that this woman takes proud in her looks and appearance. Her self-esteem is high and she isn't going to tolerate his bullshit.

From my experiences the greater a man is a sticker for getting honesty out of you. The greater your chances are in learning he is being dishonest about many things.

The second most important feature to emphasize are

the eyes. There are many ways to do this to achieve the look that best compliments your face. Play around with make-up until you find what looks best on you. Not the model in the magazine.

A good foundation and powder is a worthwhile investment. For women of color it may take shopping around to find the perfect powder or foundation to match your complexion but it is worth it. Again, learn what could be worn, when. Light powder and foundation for the day and heavier for night.

Chapter 14

<u>DRESS SEXY NOT TRASHY OR TACKY.</u>
<u>THERE'S A BIG DIFFERENCE!</u>

Another thing all the women whom all the men crowd around have in common. They aren't dressed tacky or trashy. They are dress elegant and sexy with the right amount of sexuality revealing. Leaving much to the men' imagination.

Please if you are going to go formal, go formal all the

way. It is not sexy to wear a formal dress with bare legs. Shaved or not. You might as well had arrived in jeans and t-shirt. If you're going to wear an off-shoulder or revealing neckline add jewelry that larger than a microscopic organism to show your boldness. No one's neck and shoulders are so lovely they can wear them bare without accessory.

Another thing, it is not sexy to walk around with the whole world looking at the imprint of your ass. Please wear proper underwear. It is not sexy when your dress get stuck in your ass cheeks when you sat down and everyone can see it stuck between your ass cheeks when you get up. That's tacky. That's the same as prolifically displaying camel toes. You'll get the same male's response. I know a lot of clothing comes lined but that only goes so far. If you don't know which underwears to buy call any high-end department store and describe your dress and there will a clerk there to assist you. I am saying these things for a woman to present herself respectably. Men responds to however we present ourselves. If we present ourselves as elegant and refined men rise to the occasion if he wish to talk to you. It helps weed out a lot of losers. Not only does this help you assert yourself at formal occasion but in everyday occasions also. If you dress like a hoochie you will most likely be approached like one. Just remember, men who are going somewhere in life are looking for a woman to well represent him. He isn't going to take dating you seriously if you don't take presenting yourself to the world seriously. If you dress like a fun girl that is how he will perceive you.

However, I do believe that one should dress for the occasion. There are appropriate clothing conventions we abide by for various reasons. But even if a woman respects dress codes where 'appropriate', the moment she's caught violating 'traditional social expectations' which dictate how a woman should dress – some people will question her worth, credibility, value, assume things, judge and criticize her. This is where you must learn to assert yourself and be sure of who you are and do not allow others opinion of you dictate how you feel about yourself or you won't last very long in this dating agenda. There are going to be many mean, rude, snarky people swimming around like shark when one decided they wish to pursuit a higher social economic level of dating.

Some of you may say I can not afford that look. It's not as expensive as it sound. I used the five thousand dollar dress to emphasize my point. But there are many outlets you can visit which sell high quality clothing at a fraction of the cost you would pay for some items at a discount store. These places also sells designer's make-up and jewelry. Some you can call them and order through a sales clerk if you have an idea what you are looking for and you would surprise at the steep discount that can be found on high-end items. So what if it's last season. No one has to know when you bought it. The reason I am advising this is because most women are looking a man going places with his life and have potentials.

I know we all have a right to wear whatever we want and still be respected but sorry that hasn't happened yet. Perhaps one day it will. Hopefully, we all live to see it.

Chapter 15

STOP HANDING OUT SEX LIKE LOLLIPOPS WITH NO EXPECTATIONS IN RETURN!

To the younger generation (below age forty. My own generation included.) I can't stress this enough. Stop giving away sex like it's going out of style and you're the candyman handing out lollipops at Christmas. Learn to wait at the beginning of dating to see where things are headed. You wouldn't give your car keys to a man you just met this afternoon if came over and asked for them. So why give your body to a man you don't know. It's far more valuable than your car. Waiting makes a man truly want and desire you.

There's a biological and psychological reason why he's so hot for you in the night and the next morning get up and leave never to be heard for again. Men do not appreciate that which they had to put little or no effort to get. The longer he pursue you for sex the greater his chance of falling in love with you. Eventhus, it started with him pursuing you for sex the closer he grows to you and the more attached be becomes if he is forced to wait. This is another way to weed out the players and those with other undesirable characteristics you prefer not to deal with. Those who are serious aren't going to continue to pursue for a long time. They quickly moves on to someone who will sleep with them immediately. Oftentimes saving you a lot of pain and a heartaches.

S

The Sexual Revolution may have had some good points but this wasn't one of them. Men have always wanted free flowing, non stop sex. Will at least until their desire is saturated. When it's saturated they leave us alone. The thrill is gone so they lose interest in us. It was never about love to begin with, it was all about sex. At that moment, during arousal, a large percentage of the blood from his brain is rushing to his groins so he's beside himself in releasing that pressure so he will say anything to release that pressure and once it's released and the penis is no longer in control, the blood has returned to his brain, well... it's over. This is where the Sexual Revolution ripped this power out of the hands of women. There's no known natural enzyme released in men during sex that affects their desire to be affectionate as it is in women. It doesn't affect his emotions as it does ours. So when he ejaculates, it's over. That's what all the lies are about when he promises to call or text and doesn't. You are used so he is moving on to the next person. I know this sound callous but that's how it is.

Yes, I know a man can control themselves but the society we live in doesn't hold him responsible if he doesn't. It is you who have the most to lose or gain so it is you who should be in control. It is you who can get pregnant and a child alternate your entire life not his'. A child only alternate his life if he chooses to let the child do so. Had that not been the case, the child support clerks wouldn't be over worked.

I say a man couldn't make any woman a mother he

isn't willing to make a wife but the patriarch rule says otherwise. The general rule is that it's all your fault for letting him do it. Although, I strongly disagree with the chauvinist view of things but that's the way it is. It may sound like I'm blaming women for the men' bad behavior but I'm not. I'm cautioning woman that in the real world it exists and don't live your life in a fantasy land. Fantasy land blinds you to pitfalls.

You wouldn't give anything else you own to someone after a few days or the same day of meeting him...so why would you give the most precious thing you own to someone you met for the first time in your life a few hours ago? The love lore about men falling in love after a first sexual encounter is just that__a myth. If it's true, then it must had existed before the 20th century. I can't say it can't happen but it is very rare. The man already was in love you before the act. It's said it only take a man eight seconds to fall in love. But I seriously doubt that.

S

Some may argue, "Oral sex isn't really sex." Yes, it is. If it's done right. Oh yes, it is. This misinformation is so rampart on high school and college campuses that it has even trickled down to junior high schools. It means you are no longer a virgin even if no penetration hasn't taken place. A true virgin knows a man or woman not in any sexual concept. Meaning he or she hasn't had sex with a woman or man in any shape, form or fashion.

Young ladies having oral sex is not going to land you a good life after high school or college. These guys are going to marry women who did not suck them under the cafeteria table, under the gym bench, or make out with them in cars or in a bedroom when the parents were at work. Sure, you are popular now. But wait a few year; as soon as everyone have had you, the thrill of being with you is gone. You're living your glory days now. This is why you see so many older women who were all the rave during her high school years are now with someone she wouldn't have looked twice at during her teen years. Don't let this become you. Apply yourself to getting an education for getting a man can come later in life. Real life men are far more complicated than the young adult novels you read and so are real life teenage boys. If a boy behave crude toward you. Do not pursue him. Let him be. Boys at this stage are easily persuaded by their peers and you have no idea what their peers have said. You can't change anyone's mind about you nor can you stop people from gossiping about you but one thing you can do, is make sure their gossip isn't true.

As for older women who say oral sex isn't sex, if you do it after a mere dinner date, a man is going to wonder how many men' penis you have taken into your mouth after a first date? If that's all it took to get you to suck him. He's going to view you as easy. Sure, he may add you to his sex sexacades afterward and even continue to see you for a few months but it is not going to last.

Some may say, "I got him to marry me. So, you don't know what in the hell you are talking about." Congrats. I'm happy you did. But truthfully, does he still respect you? Does he still hold you in high esteem? How does he react when you refuse to do it after marriage? Does he get angry when you refuse to perform? Respecting you goes a long way even after marriage. We all have seen married couples where a husband has no respect whatsoever for his wife. However, not in every situation she is a woman who hasn't conducted herself like a lady. Most often than not she is a lady who married a cad and needs to free herself from him and find someone who truly appreciates her.

But I'm pointing out how society has conditioned the male's mind to think of us. Most guys suffer from the Whore/Madonna syndrome. I know they say they don't but yes, they do or they wouldn't be so quick to judge us based solely on our sexual activities. A lot of men don't see women as having a healthy sexual appetite as being normal and natural. I don't give a crap what advice in women' magazines say. They don't. When trying to get someone for a life partner we still have to keep our sexuality somewhat under the wrap. I know this sounds very old fashioned but the surveys I conducted before writing this book says otherwise. I posed as a man and listed it on primarily gentlemen sites. I wasn't surprised most men still felt this way. I just needed affirmation they did.

Another thing I found that I also suspected that most men <u>do not</u> prefer a bald or shaved vagina. Some said it reminds them of a child and that's a turn off. They aren't pedophiles. The survey also said that plenty of men do not care under arm hair. It doesn't bother most men. Nor do they care about the little round belly most women have which houses our wombs. Some find it very sexy, attractive over a completely flat stomach. When looking for a mate most men do not care about the size of your boobs or butt. That when looking for a mate most men consider it a plus if you possess these attributives but on the other hand, admitted when <u>not</u> looking for a mate they looked at these as being a main attraction. So it appeared that many of the things we think they care about or main stream media has told us they do, they don't.

I found over and over the same answer, when looking for a mate. They prefer a lady. 80 percent said they wouldn't marry a woman who have slept with them too easily. The reason being is that if she slept with him so easily who else has she slept with equally as easy on the first-fifth date? Overall, men understand the power of sex and how to wield it far better than women. They know how to manipulate women far better than most women know how to manipulate a man. Mainly, because they are free to express their opinion of it without the fear of backlash whereas women are not.

Chapter 16

<u>WHEN ON A DATE DO NOT TALK ABOUT EXES, YOUR KIDS OR YOUR BOSSES. TALK ABOUT YOU. BUT LEAVE SOME MYSTERY TO YOURSELF.</u>

Don't badmouth your exes on a new date. He doesn't need to know your whole life-story on the first date to the next two months. Leave some mystery to yourself.

Let him discover who you are. Make him pursue you to learn more about you. Don't reveal every single detail about yourself immediately.

Don't cry over a broken heart. If someone else has broken your heart. Keep it to yourself. That's a complete turn off. He views it as you are still in love with your ex as to why you are crying and he is wasting his time.

Keep your personal business to yourself. Women have a tendency to reveal too much about themselves too soon. During the dating progress is the time to learn about him. Listen to what he's saying and how he says it. By listening we can learn a lot. If he criticize his exes to you he will later criticize you to someone else.

In carefully listening, learn to listen for signs that he maybe a misogynist, a narcissist, or a self-absorbed alpha male. Sometimes you can detect if he's abusive to women in what he says. Don't laugh it off if he calls another woman a bitch or says she's ugly. He may not exhibit this trait in his actions. Most abusers do not. If you hear any of these traits in the conversation. No matter how attractive he is, sadly it is best to cut your losses right then and there or suffer the consequences. Because people rarely if ever changes.

Those of you who have children, every man you date is not to meet your children. Only those who you intend to invest your life into are privileged to meet your kids. Do not spend the evening talking about your children. Do not whip pictures of your child at the dinner table. It will seems too much as if you are shopping for a new daddy for your kids. Which maybe the case; especially if you have sons but don't advertise it. If the dates grow into a relationship, he will bring this subject up. He will let you know he is in for the long haul for you and your child(ren).

If he have children by many different women and haven't married any of them. Drop him. I don't care how much money he has or how fine he is. He has serious commitment issues. Don't insert yourself in the middle of his babies' mothers' drama. It isn't worth the stress and headache. If he doesn't care about his own children don't expect him to care about yours. One of the common complaints is that none of the women were suitable for him or understood him. That's bullshit. Always keep your B.S. detector on.

Chapter 17

SAFE DATING

But also, be aware that if a man immediately during the first stage of dating shows *too* much interest in your child(ren) upon first meeting you...run. I know this isn't the case with every man. But go with your gut instincts. A date pedophile will pry the mother for information about her child or children to determine if he wish to see her again. His interest is not in you, it is in your child(ren).

In the first stage of dating, the first three months, he doesn't need to know what you do for a living. I'm saying this because there're antic people out there and most jobs are dumb asses. Believe anything someone tells them. There are sneaky snakes out there who seek to ruin you if you don't cooperate with their every demand.

For example; if he's an egoistic manic who is used to women sleeping with him on the first or second date. He has finely dined you for several weeks and still no sex. Some will seek revenge. I mean seek it in a way you never know it was them. For example; if he calls your boss and say horrible things about you most bosses are going to believe him and start treating you accordingly. I know this sounds like a petty reason to ruin someone's life but trust me. It happens everyday. Most women are taught to watch out for things such as this.

I once read of some will make women literally sick who do not meet their demands. Which is another reason I suggest waiting to get to know the person before sleeping with them. I hate to say this but there's an entire underground market that's flourishing selling these evil products to men who wish to control. No, you aren't going to find it by searching the internet. These peddlers of destruction aren't stupid enough to advertise openly. They don't want the police kicking in their door. But when doing research, I read an article that some of these diabolical peddlers frequent peek and fetish showrooms and all the men who visit them aren't there for what you may think. These are often the same places where roofies are often bought. Some uses parasites and some use germs.

Yes, that's something very scary to think about but women need not to be kept in the dark about these things. Women need to be aware there are people out there who will think nothing of ruining your health or even killing you for exercising your right to say how your life will go and they don't always come with the obvious bells and whispers as portrayed in books and movies.

Another reason a new date or boyfriend doesn't need to know your whole life story is that for all you know he maybe be an undercover stalker. If he knows where you work all he has to do is wait outside and follow you home. BAM! He's invaded your entire life. He know too much about you for safety. And having a stalker isn't fun nor cute, there's nothing anything sexy about it. It's downright dangerous and creepy. A stalker can date you and not let it be known he's also stalking you. That's his future insurance if you decide to end the encounters before he's ready to let you go. How do you think when you've broken up with someone he suddenly shows up at your job and you haven't given him your address? Somewhere along the line you gave him enough information to find you.

This is why it isn't a good idea to talk too much. One ploy some stalkers will use is telling people he is the father of your child(ren) and you are keeping him away from his kids. Most bosses aren't very bright. If they are males, sorry to say they're going to take to take the words this strange male's voice over the phone over your honest face he sees every day. And to so call get even with all the women in his life whom he feels has treated him unjustly he might take a swipe at you on the behalf of all menkind who has been mistreated by a real or imaginary evil woman. The stalker/dater might just give your out address along with lewd details about you but will never admit it shall anything happens to you.

Another common one is sending nude pictures to your job, the pictures doesn't have to actually be you. All he has to do is say they are. We live in a society where only women have to prove they are being truthful not men. The best way to tell if this has happened the boss will start behaving strangely toward you and male co-worker maybe talking about something and fall silent the moment you walk in. Or some may give you an odious look they have never given you before. Don't expect better treatment if this has happened and the boss is a woman because it's not going to happen. This past election proved that still to be true.

Another ploy is pretending to be a collection agency once he has found where you work. The boss may tell him to take the matter to your home and not bring it to your job, then he may say he brought it to your job because he doesn't know where you live. Again, your personal information will be given away as freely as the wind. I know it's illegal to give out an employee's personal information but some people can be very convincing.

The postal service often gives out information they couldn't without a clue as to who is asking. Why? I wish I knew but unfortunately people do not always think about the safety of others before opening their mouths.

Not that I have anything against cops or military men but I do not recommend them for partners. The reason being is that they have too many legal ways to harm you and there's no recourse. I know all cops and military men aren't harmful. There are many out there who are just as any other man. There are many who are good men but there are many who aren't. I'm afraid they need mates to keep them grounded just as any other man. But

I am writing about how to keep women safe during dating. Another reason I do not recommend these men is both of these jobs are very stressful and stress has a tendency to erode a relationship faster than or equal to that of monetary problems. It takes a special kind of woman who can deal with the stress and demands of these occupations. Every woman can not handle it. Studies have shown that far too often the stress spills over into domestic violence. Plus, these men have a fraternity of brotherhood and you have no way of knowing all their associates.

Therefore, it's very vital to conduct a background check on whomever you plan to let into your life. He maybe clean but you have no way of knowing that. He may actually be a nice guy and not a sociopath nor a psychopath but again you have no way of knowing these things about him. Because if he had done this before hopefully someone reported him but don't count on it. People who harm others knows very well how to cover their tracks.

Chapter 18

WHEN I SPEAK OF WEALTH I'M NOT STRICTLY TALKING ABOUT HIS WALLET.

Too often we let good guys pass us by because he isn't wealthy enough. We'd all love to find the big-hearted millionaire or billionaire who will fall in love with us but in most cases, that isn't going to happen. And from dating a few I find these men are more in love with wealth and power than they will ever be with you. Now, if this is what you want I'm not one to defer you but be prepared to deal with the fact they aren't always the most generous of men. And most are accustomed to having their way with everything. Bear this in mind that most marry women who comes from money. Meaning she is already wealthy and has attended Wharton or she is famous or has already made her money on her own. Anyway, there has to be money involved to attract big money. Or if her family doesn't have wealth they may have political clout. Because power and money goes hand in hand.

I'm not writing a book to encourage anyone to play second fiddle to anyone. Nor am I saying it can not happen but I'm writing realistically not fictionally. I say it is far better to marry a man who is in love with you and the two of you build wealth together than marry an already made millionaire.

"Wait a minute!" you maybe thinking. "I thought she just told me how to catch a millionaire????" I did. But I'm also laying out the consequences in catching one.

I have nothing against marrying a wealthy man if he loves you. I am all for it. But again, I'm writing from a realistic standpoint. Like it or not America as any other country has an unspoken class system. It's not widely talked about but it does exist. A good example of this is what happened to Gatsby in the "The Great Gatsby." Daisy didn't love her husband but Gatsby was below her social standing and she wasn't brave enough to face the scrutinizing from her social class to marry him or even send a flower to his funeral. I know this is an extreme situation but it happens far more often than we talk about. I know it's glamorized in movies that a man of substantial means meets the beautiful but regular girl and falls in love and marry her. It's a beautiful fairy tale but in reality, that rarely happens. He may often sleep with the regular girl, break her heart or even keep her for years as a mistress whom he refuses to allow to have a love life outside of himself but he very rarely marries her.

I know, I know, that burst a lot of bubbles. Like I said I'm writing about forming a meaningful relationship not a fly by night encounters. Millionaires are great for dating to see the world and experience things you normally wouldn't be able to afford but not great for falling in love with. Most are alpha males with a large egoistic personality to match. However some women can rise up to meet the criteria for such a relationship.

Now, for those of you who wish to attract this sort of

man you really have your work cut out for you. You are going to have to look like money at all times and that can become very expensive. There's no doubt about it or he isn't going to take a second glance or at least not for serious dating. You are going to have to brush up on many skills such as fine dining etiquette, conversations and such. Invest in educating yourself in many things such as fine art, classic literature, classic or fine music, expensive foods, world history and improve your language skills. This type of man is going to test your knowledge. Out of the blue, he may ask when was the Battle of Waterloo fought? He's going to expect you to be able to carry on a conversation about philosophy not the latest tabloid column.

Now comes how do you meet such a man? Most large and mid-sized cities have such things as annual charity and philanthropic balls and galas; get yourself invited to one by association if not by giving to charity or volunteering. For example if you know someone who has given a large among of money to the city, attend their social functions whenever possible. Befriend them and make it known you would like to attend a gala with them someday. Depending upon the person rather you are invited or vetted or not. But don't tell them your real reason for wanting to attend. That's shooting yourself in the foot. Like I said meeting such a man can get to be very expensive with all the requirements and such as classes, training and attending social events he may be attending. But once there, be aware you aren't going to be the only woman there on the prowl for him. The competition is stiff. Sometimes the one you attract is not the one you came for.

The best way to keep his interest after getting his attention is not to let think you *need* him or his money. These men are super paranoid about who may be after him for his money.

There's another type of millionaire who is rarely heard about for they don't advertise their wealth. That's the silent millionaire who only those close to him knows he's a millionaire. But they are harder to find than those whom everyone knows. This kind isn't likely to be found at a philanthropic party. Most are found in smaller towns and cities and in most cases.....they're already married and settled down or plan to marry the local woman whose family is old money too. His family usually has owned a local business or the house he lives in for generations is how they have been able to maintain wealth. They often they live on estates that does not appear wealthy but looks can be deceiving. They requires a different set of skills. Equestrian (horse back riding.) maybe one of them. Golf maybe another. Love of the local football or basket team he supports maybe in the equation. But with this kind, do not show any dislike or distaste for the rural way of life or you're out.

  This is the time to pull out the Saab or pick up truck and not the Mercedes. He isn't the type into flashy things and if you love shopping, this is not the man for you. This is the kind attracted to the flesh faced look and the godly woman persona. Sophistication has to hung up and left behind if you wish to attract him.

Do I recommend this? No, I do not. I wrote the instructions for those who wish to go this route in finding their millionaire. But in my humble opinion, you can have gone on twenty dates or more with men who aren't so damn choosy while trying to hook Mr. Big Stuff. I see it as too much work and too expensive for one man who may or may not be worth the effort. While there are hundreds more out there who is worth the effort and it isn't difficult to meet them.

Chapter 19

NEVER, EVER GIVE ANYONE YOU ARE DATING MONEY, YOUR CAR NOR THE KEYS TO YOUR HOME.

Yes, I am back on safety again because too often this one falls on deaf ear along with having sex too soon. With the drug epidemic in the past thirty years this practice has become quite common place. A whirlwind courtship, too soon moving in together and next thing the woman knows she is taking care of a grown man who make excuses for everything pertaining getting and holding onto a job. Some get involved with women to prevent homelessness when they have squandered all their resources on drugs. It's called a hoboromance.

The general rule of the thumb__ usually if someone wants to move very fast in a relationship there's more in it for them than for you.

Usually this man is looking a home and comfort and for someone to support him and his drug habit. Drug users can be very persuasive. The drugs teach them how to be. Sometimes this kind may work; hold down a full time job but you'll still end up supporting him for all his earnings are going into supporting his drug habit. They may occasionally help out with the bills but not enough for any real advancement. Be aware that drug abusers can become violent when high or when you refuse to hand over your money to support his habit. There's no hope for this sort of relationship unless he's willing to get help for his problem. These relationships can be costly in many ways. Court costs if he's caught using. The court cost, fines, jail time can add up to substantial amount. The traffic fines if he is caught driving under the influence and your car will get pounded and the cost to get it out can be stellar in some cities. Plus, you do not wish to deal with the elements this type of person brings into your life. Drug dealers are dangerous people.

The same applies for anyone abusing alcohol. Some people believes enough love with make them see the err of their ways. Not likely.

Chapter 20

NEVER DATE THE ANGRY MAN, HOMEBOY OR BIKER DUDE.

No matter how devilishly handsome they may be. All three of these will have you spending money you don't have to spare to bail them out of jail. All three has a very combustive personality. Which can be quite abusive and argumentative. The last two loves to hang out with their 'boys'. This can be a problem for getting and keeping a relationship going unless you are willing to let them come and go as they please. Sorry to say, that all three of these personalities are well known for being very disrespectful to women. I know urban romance glamorize the homeboy but that's all that's to it. Just a fantasy. Homeboy usually have four or five children whom he owes child support for. Usually he has gang-bangers for friends and have had several brushes with law enforcement. The same goes for **biker dude.**

The **angry man** is angry at everything and everyone. Sometimes there's a justifiable reason. If there is, you can <u>sometimes</u> work with him to learn who he truly is. Sometime the angry man feels no one have ever understood him. But if his anger is not about an injustice committed against him or a loved one which in most cases it isn't. If his anger is racial or sexual motivated get away from him because he will most likely eventually become violent. If he ever turns violent. The bet is off. He has cross the line into insanity. End it, walk away.

THE HIDER

Don't be so desperate to find someone to love you that you will accept anything that comes your way. The Hiders can pick up on this desperation a mile away. Hiders are always cheaters. They simply think you aren't good enough to be seen in public with.

Hiders will treat you well as long you do not want to go anywhere near his stomping grounds. They are never going to introduce you to their family and friends. They are never going to let you know where they live or work. A good way to tell if you are dating a hider is he can found the most romantic hidden-away spot. It's usually somewhere very few people venture. Like a park under a bridge or a national park in the middle of nowhere. He isn't going to take you to a restaurant in town for he is afraid he may encounter one of his friends and you do not meet the standard of their expectations or those of his previous girlfriends. Just as Cheaters, Hiders are good at finding little romantic places in the middle of nowhere. Hiders do not come around the holidays. It's after the holidays when you will see him again. The funny thing thus, a Hider may genuine enjoy being with you but there's something about you that do not add up to someone they want others to know they are seeing. They can be romantic and loving as long as you stay hidden.

And this definitely a no go if it's an interracial relationship. The man refuse to take you to meet anyone in his family or any of his friends after three weeks of dating. By then you could have met someone who knows him.

When conducting my interviews on the types of men before starting writing this book one woman told me a very interesting story about a Hider. She said whenever she spent the night at his place he would have her to leave under the cover of predawn so the neighbors wouldn't see her.

I asked why?

She said his neighborhood wasn't very accepting of interracial dating.

I wasn't fully understanding what she was saying. I wasn't apprehending why was she dating an obverse racist man. She told me he was a different person when the two of them were alone. He was sweet and kind until they came into town again.

I was like. "Uh hmm, that's what you call a sweet and kind man?

She lowered her eyes and head and said, "No, not really. In the end...how it ended was he started asking her to do fetish things and she wouldn't so he broke up with her."

With the Hider every story I interviewed it was the

same account again and again. Much like the woman above.

S

Widowers rarely make good partners until they are truly ready to date again. Oftentimes, well-meaning family members and friends encourages him to date to find a new companion after the death of his wife. It's best to simply offer friendship for you can't compete with a dead person.

Chapter 21

<u>WHERE DID THE BELIEF COME FROM THAT WE ARE VALIDATED BY THE MAN IN OUR LIVES??</u>

I'm warning you, this book is raw! I'm telling it like it is. If you are sensitive to certain terms, then you need to work on building up a tougher hide before you start a dating routine. Because there are lots of assholes out there who will tear your feelings and esteem down further. So be sure if you aren't suffering from being surrounded by assholes before you decide you're suffering low self-esteem. They feeling hypercritical people forces on you feels a lot like low self esteem or even depression.

But low self-esteem has a root. It's not all in your head. From the time most girls of modest to lower class means are old enough to understand what someone is saying you are being conditioned, primped and prepared for the role of a wife and mother. We are told we will meet a young man who loves us very much and we love him in return. We'll fall in love and live happily ever after. But when we reach adulthood and the prince hasn't shown up by the time we are 16-18 many of us start to become anxious. Wondering is wrong with me as to why I don't have no steady boyfriend? I was told I would one day marry and live happily ever after.

By the time we reach 24-26 we are starting to feel like a failure for having not met your prince yet because after all it was written in stone you will have met and married him. But by now you have kissed so many toads you have warts on your lips.

These emotions and expectations are a carry over from an earlier time period when women had to marry in order to survive. As little as less than a 100 years ago, in America most widows and single women lived in extreme poverty. That's where the competitiveness come from in who wins the man of substantial means. Your entire life depended upon him and his goodness or cruelty. So that was why the idea of romance was instilled in the picture. Prior to the Age of Romance, (the mid-late 1700's to the Present) there was no expectations of romance as a ground for marriage. It was all about economical advancement.

Another teaching is quite new, that a woman who marries or date a man for economical advancement is a gold digger. This didn't become popular actually until as late as the 1970's. In the early 1900's a mother didn't tell her daughter about handsome her future son-in-law was. She steered her daughter toward the man who would be able to provide well for her and didn't give a damn who she was in love with. And if that didn't work she would sic Papa on the beau. To get around Papa's word a lot of couples in love would sometime become pregnant so Papa that would have to let her marry him.

But in reality, this is not new. The American society is based upon feudal Europe. And to understand where the strain comes from you need to understand a system that was in place long before your birth.

The system was devised centuries ago so that men could stay in power. There's no other reason. It has nothing to do with you or any women. Those who devised it fully understood the power of sex. After Roman occupation in Europe many groups begin to divide into subcultures that eventually became estates and manors these estates and manors grew into nations that we know today. And the women were classified differently from the men. But like the men, medieval women were born into the second or third estate, and might eventually become members of the first by entering the Church, willingly or not. In rare cases, refusal could cost you your life.

Where did the Christian Church get idea of defining femininity? The customs of the people who taught them are not the words of God Almighty. Had that been the case Jesus Christ would have treated women as second class humans but he didn't. He treated them as equals.

One account I have always found intriguing is where the woman was brought before Jesus who was allegedly caught in the act of adultery. To any reasonable thinking person male or female; that was an oppressive law to stone someone caught in the act. All the accounts I have read of ancient stoning none of the victims were males. So who was she cheating with? And what or who gave anyone authority to dictate what someone else can do with the body God gave them? If God hadn't come from heaven chucking rocks at her and it was He who gave her the body then what authority did the patriarchal society have to do so? These accounts have always intrigued me because I'm wondering didn't those who supposedly *caught* her... have something better to do? Like go somewhere private and pray about their evil heart? Apparently, they didn't.

In feudal Europe women were categorized according to three specifically called the "feminine estates": virgin, wife and widow. There was nothing else in between. A woman's estate was determined not by her profession but by her sexual activity: she is defined in relation to the men with whom she sleeps, used to sleep, or never has slept with so being a king's daughter told her that whomever her real mother was... her father had some great affection for her. Usually infants such as herself, the mother and child was usually either killed or completely ignored or driven to destitution through shunning.

Chapter 22

WHY DOES SOCIETY GLAMORIZE ABUSIVE RELATIONSHPS?

The social idealization of abusive relationships as

romantic through literature, film, and music isn't new. Just the way it's communicated is new. What we fail to realize is that our patriarchal society benefits from the normalization of abusive behavior because it makes women idealize situations where they are forced to give up their power. For years, women have been conditioned by books, films, and music to not only accept, but to covet, relationships where they lacked any method to maintain this gendered power imbalance.

To combat this lack of power many women resorted to using sex as a weapon. Society has no one to blame but itself as to why so many women uses sex as a weapon. Anyone you leave powerless is going to find some method to gain an iota of control over their lives.

Every day we are bombarded with images, ideas, scantily dressed women and with the coming of the Internet porno is common as weeds. We see many exploitative images of women but rarely see them of men? Why is that? Men control the media and nothing in the media is designed for the benefit of women. If it is, somehow it always comes back to something to do with a man. Like I have wondered no one other than myself finds it odd that 20, 30 and 40 year old women are still fascinated by fairy tales? I'm not talking about adult fantasy romance, I mean straight up Tinkle Bell fairies with magic wand and all. This goes to show whatever we consider entertaining it has to be childish to be sociably acceptable. This is because the male dominate society doesn't want to deal with grown, assertive women. It wants to deals with little naive girls. So the media tells that it's ok and even sexy when men completely ignore us, our boundaries we are to accept it because after all it's even romantic. This very mentality toward women' partners and abusers have been allowed domestic violence to flourish.

THE ALPHA MALES

Ladies, as fine as most alpha males are and how much we love to look at them, bed them and feel their rock hard bodies smashed against us. Feel their rippling muscles. I'm sorry to say, in real life, most do not make good partners. Why? Because they must be the <u>alpha</u> in everything. The relationship must be all about them or they will find someone who is willing to make it all about them. This type of alpha male is common. Locker rooms and gyms are brimming over with them. They are great for having fun or if you want to scare off a stalker.

Now, this kind isn't totally hapless to a lasting relationship but just requires a lot of work to take his focus off himself. They can be made to fall in love with you but it is a lot of work. He falls in loves with the woman who isn't fascinated with his smoldering good looks. The woman who ignores him when he flexes his muscles, express his authority or look seductively at her as she exchanges a mere glance and dismiss him is who wins his heart. To him that's a challenge. All alpha males love a challenge. Having sex with this kind isn't going to get him. He has a long line of women wanting to have sex with him. But I do warn you with this kind do not start the dance of seduction if you want to remain free. They are the best at romance if they are trying to win a woman's heart.

If an alpha gives their heart to you they don't go away simply because you no longer want him. Or is pissed off at him. They're like lions, they mate for life. He's going to intimidate any future partners you may set your sight upon. No man in his right mind want to go up against him and he knows that. They don't give their hearts easily but when they give it, they give it all. I guess that's why there are so many romance novels written about them.

But luckily for us there are more than one type of alpha male. The Gentle Lion is what I call this type. They have all the brawn and muscles of the typical alpha male but knows when to display it. They are the handsome guy who makes every woman drool and swoon but doesn't take the advantage of their affect on women. They treat all women like a lady even if she isn't. This is a rare breed and almost extinct.

There's a myth that alphas are violent toward women. True alpha aren't. It's the fake alphas and the alpha wanna-bes who assert their authority by violence toward women and children. A true alpha male will not strike a woman back even if she hit him. But a fake alpha and an alpha wanna-bes will be. These are guys to stay away from. They are the ones who loudly proclaim their prowess in locker rooms, and everywhere else. A true alpha, no one knows who he's sleeping with for he doesn't want other men to get any ideas about his collection of women. I'm sorry for having to say it this way but most true alphas have more than one lover. I know we wish he didn't but sorry that isn't going to happen until he finds someone he loves and truly wants to settle down with.

The fake alphas and the alpha wanna-bes mostly lies about their sexual conquests and cover up their failures by saying the woman was ugly or has some other default that deflated his attention. Sadly, the media, novels and other entertainment outlets often glamorize fake or wannabes alphas for few have come across a real alpha male. When a real alpha shows up, the fakes and wannabes back down.

Another thing, all alphas aren't rippling with muscles. Some have expertise in many other areas but he is still just as much an alpha as his muscular brothers. Don't be fooled by his slim physique that he isn't an alpha. All alphas carry themselves with confidence, an assurance that borderlines arrogant. It's displayed in everything he does.

However, only you can decide the type of man you wish to spend your life with. But a word to the wise. No matter what his traits maybe if he doesn't make you happy or even tries, all the good looks in the world isn't worth the mountain of heartaches.

THE ST. JOSEPHs

Sure, there are a few sweet men out there whom your lack of confidence won't defer him. There are few out there who have been through some hardship in life and understand what it does to one's self-esteem. But this isn't your average man who will be attracted to a woman with self-esteem problems and wants to help her and lift her up. This type of man is rare and precious to the human race and again, a type nearly extinct.

But I'm writing advice for dealing with the average guy not the St. Josephs. There's no need for all this when dealing with a St. Joseph.

There are really loving, genuine, kind and respectful men out there! What we need to do is forget all the crap we see in movies. It is not real. We need to give these men a chance to love us. Give our time and bodies only to men who wants to be committed to you! And stop wasting time, energy and money on those who don't want a serious relationship.

A bad boy maybe fun for a while, I'm sure even Attila the Hun could be fun for a few dates before he started acting like Attila again. Look beyond what you see on the surface, watch his character and personality. A good hearted man is the man you want to share your heart with. Don't give yourself away too easily, don't have sex too quickly!

Some may say the time length to have sex doesn't matter. No it doesn't if you are dating a mature man who knows what he wants and isn't into playing infantile head games. But like the St. Josephs these men are few and far in between. A mature man tells you up front what he wants. Of course, all men will lie if they think you will believe them and sleep with them. But the difference is a mature man after he have lied will try to make good on the promises he made in pillow talk and not hide like a chicken whenever the phone rings. He won't avoid you even if he doesn't love you and have intentions of forming a lasting relationship with you. He will be man enough to confront you like gentleman do the things he promised he would and usually after he does them that is when it's over.

If you are looking for a lasting relationship don't have sex before you're in a loving, exclusive and committed relationship with a man who place value on your heart and body and connects with your soul.

S

Brainy, nerdy guys are not always safe to date because they are always nice people. I know there's a common perception that intelligent, nerdy guys always make excellent mates. That another myth created by Hollywood. That's not true at all. They are as any other male. You should look for personality traits. Many can be quite rude, condescending, hypercritical, insulting and downright mean. I'm not saying there aren't any nice ones but I'm warning you there are more not so nice ones than nice ones. So, don't automatically assume he's a nice nerd like Steve Urkel, because most of them of the under 40 crowd aren't. Most are rude sociopath like Sheldon. I was sorry to learn that many have a very perverted perception of women. I guess it comes from years of watching too many fantasy females online who has the two Goodyear blimps on her chest for breasts. I don't know where the sort of their feelings toward women came from but it's there.

Chapter 23

THE LOVER, ROMEO AND CASANOVO IS A LOVER OF SEX AND 'ALL' WOMEN.

This is the guy so many players try to fool you into believing that they are. But they aren't. A real player genuinely do not like women. He thrives to hurt and injure many hearts as possible. A Romeo or Casanova is the total opposite. He doesn't set out to hurt you. He let you know upfront where he's coming from. He doesn't pretend. He let you know his angle. A real Casanova genuinely loves women and would make an excellent partner or spouse if only he would love one woman. What make them so popular is a true lover or a real Romeo or Casanova doesn't distinguish women based upon traits like body shape, race, nationality. He loves all women regardless of her race, creed or national origin. That's what make this sort of man such a great lover and why so many women are attracted to him and are willing to share him. A Romeo is usually an alpha male. He treats all women with the utmost respect. He doesn't beat, abuse, belittle or use women. That's totally beneath his pride in himself. The woman who is with him at the moment knows she is the queen of the day and the jewel of his eye....at the moment. He doesn't lie to you and says he's exclusively seeing you. But when he's with you he is so good at what he does he can make you *think* he's exclusively seeing you and you alone. Some are very wealthy and some are not. Some are very handsome and some are not. But he's the guy every man secretly wants to be this guy but you are going to have give up a lot of chauvinistic bullshit to a Romeo. Another men accuses him of spoiling women with unrealistic expectations.

The odd thing about a Romeo is he doesn't true to hide you. He is confidence enough in himself to take a plain or fat girl out on town and show her to the world, even introduce her to the finer things in life. The handsome, wealthy ones aren't stuck on themselves is what attracts so many women to him. He treats the plain girl and the beauty queen equally. I have seen them take plain, sly girls under their wings and bring out the true beauty in her as no other man has tried to do. These are the guys that boost women confident not tear it down. He's the type of guy whatever he does for a woman he isn't expecting repayment. Those whom he dates knows she doesn't have to put out until or if she's ready. He doesn't pressure her. He will tell a woman to never allow anyone to treat you lesser than the way I've treated you.

Now, the positive side about dating one is once you've experienced a real Casanova all other men will become pale in comparison and you look for a man who will treat you how he treated you which is very romantic and like you were the only woman on earth.

This kind of man can be your best male friend. He will give you advice on other men and who to dump and who to keep. Unfortunately, he's the guy every man hates with a burning passion. He's the perfect man all except one thing. He's a manwhore. He isn't going to be true to one woman. So do not fall in love with him. That's why a model of his personality trait serves as the ideal lover and is used in so many romantic novels, movies and etc. He loves women and usually one day fall in love with someone and when he does he leaves all the others behind.

So you may wonder with all these terrific attributes is the Romeo worth the wait? I would say he's not. It's better to move on to find a man who is willing to be exclusively yours. For there's no guarantee you will one day win his heart and become his lady love. Which is why I advise if you still wish to maintain contact with him; it better to be his friend.

Chapter 24

THE ROAMANCER

The **roamancer** is just what he sounds like. A flighty person. Someone who is merely in love with the idea and concept of being in love not the person he's dating.

They possesses many of the traits of a Romeo but they will lie to you. They roams from one woman to the next. The dating or courtship is usually a whirlwind of romance and activity for a short while and then suddenly or abruptly stops. Giving you no clue as to why. Unlike a Romeo, a roamancer will make you believe you're exclusive. He will do all the things that a man should do for a short while and it ends without a clue as to why. Some will even promise marriage and speak of planning a future within weeks of starting to date you but they are as flicker as butterflies. Be aware, some roamancers operates in burglary rings. They send in the best looking one to do the "getting-close-and-personal." When they disappear so will all your valuables.

Chapter 25

THE HYPERCRITICAL GUY

Avoid him like the plague. If you didn't have a low self esteem problem...oh yes, you will definitely have one if you date him long enough. He's going to criticizes every single detail or every little thing about you. Things you hadn't notice. He will point them out. Nothing about you will ever be good enough for him. He strives and lives on public opinion. If anyone else thinks something is off, wrong, or bad about you he won't hesitate to let you know it and gives you tips on how to improve whatever he or others think is wrong with you.

Too bad, too many women view this kind of behavior as a man being concerned and loving when that isn't his agenda at all. You must be exactly as he approves or he will nag you bald. Nag you until you change into someone you don't recognize anymore.

But the really sad part about being with a man like this. Even after all the weird ass changes to appease him you may still end up being dumped because he's a rigid perfectionist. And no one is perfect.

Chapter 26

<u>JUDGE A MAN BY HIS TREATMENT OF OTHERS</u>

There many indicators of mature a man or a St. Joseph. One of the primarily ones to watch is how he treats the women in his life such as his mother, sisters, and other female relatives. If he treats them horrible then he will treat you worst.

And second indicator is how did he have treated his ex wives or girlfriends before they broke up? Don't automatically believe him if he speaks negatively about them. Because when break up with you he will say the same to the next woman. Try to learn if the every break up her fault or his'? That's important because habits in relationships are the baggage a person carries with them from one relationship to another until they mature enough to realize if they keep fucking up they are going to keep having the same problems in every relationship. Sadly, with both men and women, some never grow up and realize this. It's easier to blame the other person than to look at the person in the mirror.

Thirdly find out if he has any female friends or if he believes that men and women can not be friends without sex being in the equivalent. If he has them find out how he treats them? Does he treat them the same as he does his male friends? Or he treats his male friends better and treat the females one as someone he merely tolerates for whatever reason.

The fourth one, the next one is very important. How does his male friends treat women? The reason this is so important is after a boy reach his teens his male friends have a lot of influence on his behavior. If hangs with guys who has no respect for women, then most likely he doesn't either. Or else he wouldn't hang out with them. If these friends have more influence on him than you. Then the relationship isn't going to last.

Fifth but one of the most important of them all. Always, I mean always watch how his father treat his mother? Is his father abusive to his mother? Are they married or have been married? I know this isn't always a clear indication of how one will behave but if the father doesn't see fit to marry the man's mother. Most he likely the son won't see any reason to marry any woman either.

I am fully aware that some sons of abusive fathers become the best husband and father any woman could ask for after seeing the suffering of his mother, he declares he will never treat a woman so horribly.

Another indicator, ask him to associate with male relatives, or male friends you trust. Men know other men better than we know men just as we know women better than men know women. How does your father or other male relatives feel about him? Do they think he's a good person?

Be prepared to listen even if you think they are wrong. I know with some brothers and fathers no guy is good enough for you but if they constant to say the same thing eventually you will see what they saw in him.

BE SURE HE'S THE MARRYING KIND.

Before investing time and energy in man, even a St. Joseph you need to find out if he's the marrying kind? All of, even St. Josephs aren't the marrying kind. Some has been married and was burnt and others may have seen no purpose in marriage. No amount of time is going to change his mind until he's ready to marry.

I'm not talking about the fiance who is trying to achieve a goal in life like getting his college degree before marriage. It would be senseless to get married when one isn't financially stable enough to do so.

Which reminds me, I once attended the wedding of a couple who were both homeless and living on the San Bernardino beach. I was at the beach with my husband and child and the local charity organization sponsoring the wedding invited us over as guests. But I thought it was odd after the ceremony and reception of fruit punch and cake they went back to their tent on the beach. They gave new meaning to sex-on-the-beach. I thought someone could be finding them a resident rather than giving them a wedding. We stayed at the hotel for five days and they were still on the beach when we left. But I guess they were happy.

Chapter 27

IT DOESN'T TAKE FOREVER AND TEN YEARS FOR A MAN TO DECIDE IF HE WANTS TO MARRY YOU

It doesn't take years of dating for a man to decide if he wants to marry you. He has usually already decided that after the first or second date. Although, he may not propose quite that soon but it is on his mind. It's a myth proliferated by society that it takes men years to be sure. No, it doesn't. Even five year old boys know that's a lie. That's why he gives the little girl in his kindergarten class candy and tell her she will someday be his wife and won't leave her alone.

After six months to a year if he hasn't made any serious attempts to propose to you or talk about a future together or cringe everytime you mention a commitment then he isn't going to. If everything is comfortable; why could he? So, it's time to move on. He's wasting your time and keeping you from someone who is looking for the same things you are.

Chapter 28

DON'T OVER LOOK THE NICE GUYS FOR SHALLOW REASONS.

Unfortunately, most women tend to overlook the good guys for the same shallow reasons men overlook the nice girls and women. We are as guilty as men of selecting a mate with more looks over brains. Just as guys often choose the woman with the largest female attributes such as breasts and asses, we often overlook the St. Josephs because he isn't exciting enough or muscles are big enough or he doesn't make enough money.

STOP WASTING TIME WITH RELATIONSHIPS THAT AREN'T GOING ANYWHERE

This is one of the major complaints of females of couples cohabiting together. The scenario usually goes something like this; she moved in about one-five years ago. The couple has 1-2 two children but he still refuses to pop the question. Sorry, ladies but it look our mothers and grandmothers were right when they said, "Why buy the cow when you can get the milk for free?" The reason he hasn't popped the question is that he is leaving his options open for someone he considers more compatible than you. It's doesn't take anyone five years to make up their mind about a relationship. I once watched a show where the couple had been dating for 18 years and finally got married after their daughter finished high school. I watched everyone make a big deal over he finally asked her to marry him after dating her since they both were 17 years old. Sooo, it took someone eighteen years to figure out they loved you but took only eight seconds to figure out they wanted to screw you?

Some people say give him the ultimate and put a time limit on it. But I disagree. I say they have already spoken their true feelings so believe them. This is nothing but another example of wasting your time. I believe as Mark Twain said, "Never allow someone to be your priority while allowing yourself to be their option."

Chapter 29

<u>WHAT REALLY ATTRACTS A MAN.</u>

If you want to know what attracts and turns the heads of men in your path? It all depends upon the man and what he's looking for. Different men are attracted to different things. But the number head turner is confidence. Self-assurance. It shows in everything you do.

As I wrote in the beginning of the book men aren't as easily turned off by certain things like a little hair in certain areas or the notion that everything must be perfectly presented as the glamor magazines laden and designed to sell us produces as the so-called experts would have us to believe. True, there are some who are like that but these are usually very hypercritical, shallow men who would be a waste of your time.

Those totally ruled by superficial, materialistic world are what we are trying to get away. The type of men who are solely attracted to a woman's physical appearance. Although, well grooming plays a vital role in attracting a man. We are trying to return to an earlier time when one could find men attracted to your soul. Men who wanted to get to know you as a person. Not simply as a sex buddy.

I'm hearing more and more men talk about since sex has become so plentiful love is harder to find. Well, they are the reason they can't find love. Some need to lower their expectations to a real person and realize no one is perfect not even themselves. And you can't find love bed hopping. The reason they can't find love is they aren't looking for it. Women are using you for sex the same as you are using them. Most women are looking for men with something to offer than a roll in the sack and aren't going to invest her heart into anything less. Women discuss among each other who is good in bed and who is not. Sooo, if one woman after another approach you for sex. Buddy, your name maybe on the bathroom wall.

Chapter 30

WHERE ARE THE MEN?

Men are everywhere. Grocery stores, libraries, bars, restaurants, websites, on the streets, etc. In large cities it is harder to attract a man merely on the streets, but it can be done. You can attract a perfect stranger. At first watch him for a few minutes first to try to determine whether he maybe a nutjob who is going to later stalk you if things don't work out. Then walk up and say hello and introduce yourself. You don't have give a total stranger your real name. It's safe not to. If he's interested give him a way to get a hold of you. Email addresses work just as well as phone numbers and are much safer. I find midsize towns and social events are the best places. In large cities everyone is impersonal and antisocial for very good reasons. Small towns aren't good. They maybe for a few people but not for everyone and if you are looking for an upward mobility man. Most, if from a small town have long ago left so you may have to do like the birds. Go to greener pastures.

HOW TO SEDUCE WITHOUT BEING OBVIOUS THAT'S WHAT YOU'RE DOING.

All you have to do is look him confidently and seductively in the eyes. Don't lower your eyes even if he frowns a little at first, wondering why you are looking at him. I don't mean the oversexed seduction as portrayed in movies such as saying dumb shit like "I want you so bad." He might think you are hooker. But a mere smile with your eyes is all it takes to get him to stop on the streets. Hold eye contact with him. I promise you even a stranger will come to you.

For those who aren't bold enough for that a modest glance will do. Let him catch you watching him and look away several times, if he's interested he will come over.

What do you talk about once you get him at your side? Being observance, all men like praises. If he's wearing a nice tie, tell him you think it looks nice on him. This is where enlightening yourself comes into play. Usually everyone has heard something about the latest events.

Don't go into heated issues like politic or religion when striking up a conversation for the first time. Something as simple as the weather will do.

But if he makes lewd comments. Don't excuse them or smile them away. Walk away. He has already told you why he came over.

If you are at a party and there's a man you wish to talk to or date. Walk pass him and glance at him and keep walking. Put sway to your hips and believe me. If he's alive. He will look. And if he doesn't, try it again. Some can be kind of dense. After the second time if he doesn't catch the hint and follow then leave him alone. He isn't interested. Move on to someone else. Moving on to someone is more likely to make him sit up and pay closer attention.

If you are at a park and see someone you wish to talk following the same as at a party. But it can be easier for he is usually outside reading or involved in some out door activities. Approach him about what he is reading or doing. Yes, I know there are some rude men out there but listen to your instincts before approaching him. After a few minutes of conversation invite him to a nearby stand or cafe for a drink. Never go to a bar. That will give him the wrong impression of you. If he declines, then move on. It's hard to know in public what's a stranger's reason for declining an invitation. Don't feel obligated to disclose personal information about your-self simply because you invited a guy for a cup of coffee. All that comes later if the two of you decides to go a date. Give your date phone number to a stranger not your real phone number nor address.

Well, if he's gay then nothing is going to work on him.

I do not recommend dating bosses or co-workers. There an old saying: "Do not piss where your bread and butter is." Meaning there's always a possibility of a bad date or bad break up and you shouldn't bring your personal life to work. It's difficult to go back to the way things were with those you work with after dating or having sex with them.

But the easiest and surest ways of to attract men is project an air of confident. Keep your appearance attractive and modest. No skimpy clothing, you do not wish a man to see everything you have to offer from a mere glance. Because in reality sex is his sole reason for dating you. Why could he ask you on a date when he already see every thing he wants to see with your merely walking down the streets?

SOMETIMES YOU HAVE TO MOVE TO FIND THE TYPE OF MAN YOU ARE SEEKING.

Some believe you have to go some places to look for them. I find that to be true depending on where you live. Some areas literally have no eligible men. What I mean by eligible is men? I mean men who know how to date, aren't in a relationship, aren't married, aren't besieged by drugs or alcohol, aren't gay, has some form of gainful employment, who don't have I-like-hitting-women syndrome, who aren't the father of half of the town with 10 baby mamas. Some areas literally have no men who don't fall into one of these categories.

One thing never to do, is be the side woman or outside woman. That's a dead end from the start. He may treat you well, he may pay your bills, he may do all the things that a man could do but there's many things he'll never do. Take you home to his family or spend the holidays with you or make a commitment to you.

For those who have read only a few pages of this book and believe I'm a man basher, you haven't read far enough into the book yet. I highly suggest to you ladies nothing turns a man off faster than man bashing. They know there are some men out there who are complete jerks. But don't remind them on this on a date if he hasn't given you a reason to.

EMPOWER YOURSELF

Empower yourself. No one else can do this for you. This is something you must do for yourself. Take the time out to broadening your knowledge, learn new skills and hone your communication skills. It won't always lead you to finding the right man. But it will help build your self-confidence. Believing in yourself and knowing your worth will give you confidence and feel good about yourself that will enable you to select a mate that is best suited for you. It gives you courage to wait, so that you do not make a life alternating decisions out of fear you will never get the chance again so you better settle for what you can get.

OVERLY PICKY MEN ARE A WASTE OF TIME

Do not waste your time on extremely picky or very selective men. We all have certain physical attributes we are attracted to. But this goes far beyond that. I'm talking about the kind of man who will only seriously date someone with certain narrow attributes. The list is so long it would take an entire book to write them all. But for an example some only dates blondes, women with huge bust-lines, women with flat rear ends, with certain birth marks, women with tiny feet, etc. I'm sure you get the picture.

We all have preferences we'd like in a mate. But often find and chose someone with none of the attributes we find attractive because we fall in love with who they are not how they look. Again, that's not what I'm talking about. I'm speaking of the kind of person who would break up with someone he loved all because she didn't fit his strict list of requirements.

How would you know you are dating someone like this? A good indicator is who and what he watches on a woman when with you. This kind is easy to spot for if a woman pass with these required statures he isn't able to resist watching her. Usually they are only dating you to kill time until they find the woman they want. But in the meantime, if you continue to date him he will ask you to make changes like dye your hair, have breast implants, or criticize these features about you. Don't make any changes for this person for they are going to be gone in a few months or weeks anyway. When you discover you are merely a rest stop get out. Don't waste your time getting out of the dating routine because there will never be a relationship and he is in-between his types and the moment he finds another who suits his taste you won't hear from him again.

Let face it some men have so many requirements that it's exhausting. So many that even the Holy Mother of God wouldn't be able to meet them all. They would find some fault with even her. The reason I say do not waste your time is while you are keeping him company while he waits for someone who meets at least half of his requirements the guys who truly wants to date you are out there passing you by.

RESPECT, DEMAND IT.

Yes, I'm back on respect again because lack of it is a major culprit in today's dating. When I was single I was very much pursued by the opposite gender. So I must had been doing something right. I know I owe it a lot of it to my self confidence and knowing my worth. Never settle for anything less than your worth.

Too many women do not know their worth or throw it all away believing they can earn a man's love. But sadly, that's the opposite. Always demand respect. If a man can not and will not respect you don't expect him to ever love you.

Chapter 31

THE BUTT GIRL

Respect goes beyond what goes on in public, it extends to what happens privately also. Men will test your virtues even after you agreed to have sex with him. Anus sex is a quickest way to make a man walk, men do not do anything for the woman they can fuck in the ass.

I do not know why but they don't. Everyone knows men do not marry the butt girl as they'll call you once you agree to have anus sex. I know there's going to be a lot of outcry about this one. But who has the diamonds and jewelry to prove this true, me or you or the man who wants to poke you in the butt? I do, so I know what I am talking about.

I wrote this because unfortunately, not everyone is enlightened enough not to apply labels and some men have preconceived ideas about certain sexual activities and positions. Like it or not, some people still judge, criticize and condemn women for embracing their sexuality. What makes me so mad and quite honestly, fucking angry – is that there is so much self-hatred in this world. Women who truly do not like themselves. There are so many women who suffers from body-image issues, low self-esteem and depression. Why are we trying to bring people down and shame women for embracing themselves, or for showing an ounce of confidence? It's hard enough to love yourself in a society that constantly tells you that you're not good enough. Which is why I keep recommending building self confident. This way other's opinion will affect you less. Feminism isn't about policing other's people's bodies, it's the exact opposite. I do not agree with this silliness but I am warning it does exist and be on the lookout for it.

Positions like anus sex is for once you've married him not before. The marital bed is where you experiment and let your desire run loose. Not before. Too many women make this mistake. Thinking it will excite him to the point of falling in love with her. But it will not. Even after you become lovers do not let down your guard until you have said "I do". I know this sounds old-fashioned and passe but if you be too big of a freak in the bedroom he will view you as promiscuous. Never, ever get yourself labeled, "The Butt Girl" or the "Bottle Girl"

Chapter 32

SAY NO TO BONDAGE

This is another relationship killer. I don't care what the media says. They can make all the movies and write all the books they wish to about it. Never accept any type of bondage as a part of your sexual activities. There's nothing sexy or healthy about letting someone beating the hell out of you nor tying you up. If you are dating someone and learn he's into weird bondage sexual activities, it is far better to move on. It's best to kiss the chances of it developing into something more. Goodbye.

Chapter 35

NO SEX PICTURES

Sending or texting him sex pictures is not appropriate behavior. It makes you seems desperate and lonely. Even if you are, he doesn't need to know that. Men equivalent 'desperate' with being clingy and clingy means this is the woman whose pictures he will share with his friends. This is how so many embarrassing pictures ends up on the internet. There used to be a male's revenge site where naked pictures of ex-girlfriends and wives found their final resting place. Don't give anyone pictures that can land in this dump.

Chapter 33

MR. CHEAPO IS USUALLY MR. CHEAPERO

There's another reason I say do not accept so called cheap romantic dates in the beginning of your seeing him. If he barks at taking you out to dinner, buying you gifts and always suggest a cheap place or a hideaway place to eat. Drop him. A man who want you is never ashamed of you. He wants the world to know how much he cares you.

Usually he is cheating if he keeps it up after several months of dating. This is a good indication he's already in a committed relationship and doesn't want the wife or girlfriend inquiring about missing income as to why you are having lunch under the Brooklyn Bridge in the park.

If has proven to be single but yet he never remembers you for Valentine's Day, your birthday, nor Christmas. Why are you with him? No, love isn't based upon what he can afford to buy you but a man who loves you will find a way to do things to show his appreciation of you. Another good indication of how things will go; if he doesn't do anything before he moves in with you or marry you do not expect him to do anything afterward. Because a person is on their best behavior during courtship and what you are seeing is his best.

Chapter 34

__NEVER TAKE CARE OF GROWN ASS MAN__

I can't say this one enough because so many people (women) are engaged in this practice in hope that it turns into some serious. It's one of the dumbest thing I have ever seen some women do. Totally support their husband or boyfriend and he does nothing. He takes her to work everyday and keeps the car. Why do he needs a car if he does nothing all day? And just what do you think he's doing all day with it if he isn't working? He's driving around town with other women and his friends. Make him get a job even if it's nothing but flipping burgers at a local fast food restaurant.

Chapter 35

THE PERFECT GUY

First all, there's no such thing as a perfect guy, he only exists in two places, in fairy tales and the bible. The more perfect he seems the more he's hiding. Mr. Perfects are good at hiding things. They are a lot like the Hiders except they hide character flaws until you have invested your heart, mind, body and soul into the relationship and that's when their true color shines. Mr. Perfect is more concerned about his appearance to the community than he is with his treatment of you. That's how he has been getting away with his dirty deeds all these years. No one believe he's capable of beating you black and blue. Because he's usually the pillar of the community type. Usually Mr. Perfect has a long track record of abuse toward women. Mr. Perfect will blame you for everything that goes wrong. If he suffers impotency... it's all your fault. Never mind there maybe an underlying medical problem.

If anything is out of order in a household or his life, it's your fault and your fault usually means a beating or withholding of affection.

Mr. Perfect is a very manipulative and can be dangerous person. They will do anything to get their way. Some has been known to kill and have gotten away with it. All because no one believed he was truly capable of such heinous crime.

A good sign a guy may be a Mr. Perfect...outward he may appear to have it all together; terrific job, good looks, genteelly, romantic, and thoughtful. Who wouldn't want a guy like that?! Outwards he is a great catch but interesting enough... he has never had a lasting relationship. It's virtually impossible to find any of the women he previously dated. It's like he has a clean slate in the dating world.

Mr. Perfect will slowly start to take over your life. Demanding, politely at first to know your every move before moving to forcefully demanding that you obey his orders and report your whereabouts at all time to him. If not men such as him can tell very violent.

Chapter 36

NO PUBLIC DIRTY DANCING

When out dancing and having a good time, for the love of all womanhood do not twerk hm. Or you will dance his respect for your right out the window. Sure he loves it. Because he is deciding how the date will end. Dance respectful, don't let him grab your ass or breasts in public. That within itself tells you all you need to know about how much he respects you and what his intentions are in the future because a man who want you do not wish to call other guys' attentions to any parts of you. They are possessive about other guys looking at these parts of you as dogs are pertaining his bone.

Chapter 37

ORAL SEX, I THINK NOT.

I know, I'm taking all the fun out of dating and sex. But do you want to get married or not? Oral sex is another no-no, I don't care what they say, but the moment you suck him he has already lost some degree of respect for you. I know this is going to be another outcry. Some are going to ask me am I speaking from the Victorian Age? No, I'm not. I'm speaking of how a man's mind actually works not the bullshit he and the media tell you. Some may ask you have you ever performed either of these acts? Say no, because if he asks. He's testing to see what you are made of. He's trying to decide if you are worth his time after the sun rise.

To show he cares about pleasing you even after you have say no, he'll perform it on you and in most cases, won't ask you again.

S

Listen to what he says, if he calls and instead trying to serenade you he blurts out he's horny and want to fuck you and just how hard he wants to do it. Hang up the phone or don't text back for that's all you are going to get. You aren't going to get a tender session of love making. There's a big difference between making love and having sex. Any man can have sex but it takes a real man who cares about you to make love to you. Some may call back and apologize but that tells you a lot of where the relationship was headed.

Chapter 38

THE MISANTHROPIST MYGONGIST

If he refuses to respect you then there's nothing you can do to change his feeling about you or women in general. Because most men like that genuinely do not like women and feel all women are disingenuous and manipulative. Don't waste your time with such a man. You are only going to get hurt, put down, and in some cases, a beat down. They are a misanthropist. Some has been socially conditioned to be so and never matured enough to grow beyond the cave man complex. There's a common misconception that a misogynist does not like sex with women. They love sex with women as much as any man. It's females as a gender they don't like. If we would detach our vaginas and give them to these types of men they would be very happy. But unfortunately for them we can't do that.

There's a hidden type of misanthrope, the kind that detest a woman the moment he has an orgasm. He finds her disgusting and wants nothing more to do with her.

This kind can be dangerous and will sometimes kill or harm women after or during sex which is why I advise against certain sexual activities like choking, spanking, bondage, and etc. For if he has this hidden tendency it will surface during the violence of these practices. No, I am not talking about rapists. You know they are violent. I'm talking about hidden misanthropes. They can be sweet, charming and even loveable until you agree to sleep with him. When it's over that's when he despises you. More men have this problem than any will ever admit it. This account for perhaps 50% of the suddenly dropping you after sex scenarios.

Being a misanthrope is the OFTEN a cover for a 'player'. Players genuine do not like women. They don't see them as human beings less alone their equal. That's how they can so easily move from one woman to another. Because players don't wait for sex. None do they want sex most of the time. It's about the conquest. If you don't put out he move from woman to woman until he finds someone who will.

Another hidden type of misanthrope is a **racist misogynist**. He will sleep with women of races other than his own but rarely will marry anyone outside of his own race. Because those not of his race are the only women he have been taught to hate. He hasn't been taught to hate women of his own race as to why those of his own race never see this side of him. The racist misogynist can be kind and loving as long you do not demand to be seen publicly with him or some has been known to marry outside their race but the marriage falls apart due to constant criticism. It's one of the sadness things to see is a racist man trying to be a lover. You can't be a true lover unto women if you're any of these things. You are merely a fucker. There's a big difference between a fucker and a lover. A true lover or a real Romeo or Casanova doesn't distinguish women based on these traits. He loves all women regardless of race, creed or national origin. That's what make this sort of man such a great lover and why so many women are attracted to him.

Chapter 39

<u>THE LOVER</u>

This is a term widely used but many people have no idea what a lover is. It isn't someone merely having sex with you. That's someone who simply fucked you.

A lover loves women. Period. He's what many men strive to be but very few achieve it. Too many women mistaken a player for a lover and get burnt. Women love a lover because they know he's usually truthful with them unlike a player who waste their time playing infantile mind games. A lover doesn't distinguish between women based upon race, shape or size of body parts, and other pettiness. A misanthrope does that. But a lover isn't the man to give your heart to. Because just as he is wooing you; he's wooing many others. Depending on what you are looking for. If you are looking for simply sex, fun, a good time then a lover is the man to seek out. Some will shower you with expensive gifts and trips but do not expect a commitment. Most lovers will tell you they aren't interest in a commitment and if you are. Then leave the table. You aren't going to change him. Your falling in love with him isn't going to change a thing.

Chapter 40

SEX TOO OFTEN LOSS THE FLAVOR

Another thing I found as a no, don't do. Do not give a man sex every time he wants it. Make him desire you and want you, not mere lust after you. Some argues that he could have sex whenever he wants it. No he couldn't. People get anything whenever they want it and doesn't have to put forth any real effort to get it, they soon take it for granted or lose interest. Too many women are too afraid he's going to leave and seek sex elsewhere if she withhold herself from him. If he does, then let him go. He was never yours to have and to hold to begin with. They don't seem to realize women can sit on their pussies for years without sex, so it's men who have to do what women want. Not the other way around.

Some even argue that withholding sex when your man let you down or displease you and reward him with hot sex if he make you happy is manipulative and very honesty. Claiming that this very idea is why men think all women are insincere and artful. I can tell you whomever thinks that has never been married and probably will never get married.

Call it whatever you would like but sex is the only leverage a woman has and if she gives it up every time he ask or demand then she has given up all her power and when a woman become powerless in a relationship in many cases the man starts to lose respect for her. By nature, men are chasers and hunters. If we do not make them work for the sex they get they start to wonder if she didn't make him work for it she probably doesn't make any man work for it. Like it or not that's how their mind works.

I know it's popularly portrayed in movies, songs and romance novels that the guy not having to work for it but still falls madly in love with you after buck wild sex. That only happens if he was already in love with you before he slept with you.

No, it is not manipulative or dishonest. That's what is called wielding the power of sex. Think about the reason you are upset? Was he being inconsiderate, manipulating your emotions for his own endgame? And how will he ever improve his bad behavior if you reward him for it with red hot sex?

Chapter 41

SECURITY OR LOVE?

I hate to sound callous of the heart but in America and the Western world we believe that all marriages must be based upon love in order to work. I too, believes that. But I know that isn't always a reality. And for a long time, it wasn't a reality, nor an expectation even in the Western world or America. Actually, the sole idea of marrying for romantic love is something that didn't became a common practice until the last hundred and eighty years. Before then, often friends and family members arranged for the couple to meet based on his finances and the couple's compatibilities.

Often the couple grew to love each other after marriage not before. Today's women do not need the security to the same degree as women needed it in the 1800's – mid-1900's but it is a vital part of a marriage. Money is the single most reason couple argues. And if financial security is no big deal as the modern agenda teaches then what are people arguing about? The reality is that his love may give you such a thrill but it can not pay your bills.

Not that many will admit this but this practice is still quite common among the extremely wealthy as to why they usually only marries another extremely rich person. Their is more of a hushed caste system being maintained than a financial agenda as the reason why.

Selecting a partner is an investment in your most important agenda. Your life. A partner make it or break it. Depending on who he is as to why the choice should never be taken lightly.

Chapter 42

COMPLIMENT YOUR MAN.

Just as women men needs reassurance from time to time also. So do men. So, compliment your man with positive activities and praises, this builds up his self image and confidence! When he is happy so are you. There will be arguments and more peace, I promise an unhappy man can make you miserable as he is!

If he does something wonderful, tell him. If he doesn't do something so wonderful. Tell him. But tell him as you are speaking to an adult not as if you are a mother scorning a disobedience child. He'll only resent and resist your every word and start acting like a strong-headed, disobedience child. A loving man will listen and not become angry or ignore you. Tell him know he has a support system in you. A couple in harmony has far better sex than a couple who hold resentment toward each other. If he's rewarded with hot sex when he does well. He will drastically improves. Remember, I'm talking about a solid relation here. This is not going to work with a fly by night boyfriend.

Chapter 43

TECHNOLOGY AND SEX

In today's age of technologically too often females are easily acquirable, when accession should be limited to the opposite sex but is not. This create a greater tendency to cheat and can destroy a relationship.

Learn how to properly manage yourself via text messaging, e-mailing, and of course, social networking sites such as Facebook, Twitter and etc.. Internet dating can be fun but if you feel you have been duped, played, etc., you need to step back and look for red flags. I advise this for both men and women. There are con artists out there who are very good at playing others with love-games and you need to be able to detect such types. They've been doing this for years and gets away with it because they're experts at the game. This game can get very costly when you start sending money to a loved one you have never met. Usually these people will make excuses as to why you can not meet them in person. Usually they are conning more than one person. Many of the nude pictures you see they aren't there just for show. It's a con. To talk to the woman behind the photo requires payments.

Not everyone online is out to get you but everyone needs to be aware that these personality types do exist. Detecting BS is a great start when dealing with someone you haven't met. Sometimes that's all you have to go on. Because dating profiles may not be accurate.

Always treat others online as you wish to be treated. Even as knowledgeable as I'm about men, when I was in the dating world I tried to use my sapience to the best of my abilities and not lead others on. Once you acquire the needed confidence needed to know your worth don't let it swell your head. Unfortunately, too many people do. But don't ever forget to treat others how you'd like to be treated. If you're communicating with someone but finds someone else who suit you better, make sure you state it kindly to the first person you were talking to. Don't leave a person hanging on to hopes. That is cruel in real life and online. Don't hide behind a screen as a cover for your cowardice or callousness.

Chapter 44

<u>PREDATORY PLAYER</u>

This type of player is different than the regular run-of-the-mill player. This type of player is often mistaken for a lover from how sweetly he can play the game. But online and off every woman or teenager who is dating needs to know about the games these men play. Some believe some players are harmless and easy to pick out that they are just after sex. That's true, some are harmless and easy to pick up on their motive. They don't stick around.

But there is a darker, more sinister side to this, there are some who are more insidious & predatory. They are experts at their game, they'll seduce you not only out your dignity but your money as well. They will mislead by outright lies, deceive, manipulate and use women until they cause serious destruction that some women never recover from. That's their goal, to destroy you. Consequently, every woman needs to take the time out to learn the difference between them. What to look for in these types of men. One clue, is they are like Mr. Perfect, too good to be true. They know what women want and like in a lover. They use sex as a weapon. This is the kind of man who will give you all you need for maybe six months. They have a time span just as regular player. Let's say he gives you six thousand in six months. Well by the seventh month he's going to create a sod story needing seven thousand and if you are hesitant he will say, "Baby, you know I'm good for paying you back. In a few months, you are going to be mine's any way." Although, he has no intentions of marrying you or even firmly establishing a relationship. So don't do it.

Everything he invest in you he's going to retrieve it twice over and everything you are reluctant he will remind you of his love for you and what he did for you in the beginning of the relationship.

This type of player works hard to make you emotional dependence upon him. He plays minds games. He's hot one moment and cold the next. Or can even be abusive and if you dig deeper you may even find where he once was or still is a pimp. I kid you not. That's where he learned the tricks of his trade. Through the world of prostitution.

Pay close attention to feelings that things aren't adding up. Don't let him cause you to dismiss your natural female instincts as whiny or frivolity. Beware of the *'perfect' guy* and *the 'perfect'* relationship that moves too quickly and unfolds too easily. This how the predatory player starts out. In the beginning, nothing is too good for you. This is the bait. Within months the behavior start to shimmer down. He starts needing things you have no idea why he needs it. And can make it sound like a matter of life and death if he doesn't get it. So eventually you may end up taking out loans and second mortgages and may not know the reasons why?

In consequence, watch to see if his action correlates with his words. If they do not. Then he's lying. Get the hell out of the relationship while you still have some sanity left. Because this guy isn't going to stop manipulating you until you are useless to him. Know this, a guy who is genuinely interested in a relationship is willing to put forth a real effort to build something healthy and lasting. Not one create a house built of bricks of lies. A real man will listen and try to soothe your concern and fear. Not amplify them. A man truly interested in you help solve problems not create them with lies and manipulations. He respects you and is proud to be with you, your opinion matters to him and in most cases, he's open and lucid with his intentions.

Chapter 45

YOUR DAY IS MONDAY, HER DAY IS TUESDAY

A player is improbable to commit any real effort in a woman, to him she is just a wayside station. For he's seeing other women and they are all on a schedule. He has assigned you a certain day of the week and you won't see him until your day has come. Get out if he refers to you as a 'special friend,' never as his girlfriend and you haven't been introduced to his friends, family or even acquaintances or whenever you confront him with profession or promises made he claims he can't recall them or didn't say that so surely you misunderstood. According to him there's always an excuse as to why he can not do certain things.

Chapter 46

THE PATHOLOGICAL LIAR

We are all aware that men lie about love. That's nothing new. But there some who not only lie about love to get sex, but nothing comes out their mouth is true. If he tells you that he loves you and act otherwise, then he's lying. They lie about everything. Meaning everything from their job to where they are from; they lie about everything from their real name to their real age, occupation, their status of being single or married. The reason it's a red flag is that this step isn't necessary for men. He doesn't have to take personal safety into the same perspective as a woman does. So why is he lying? To manipulate and turn the tables to his advantage.

Some of us have fallen in love with our **sweet little liar.** These aren't exactly men who lie for destructive reasons; to hurt and harm you. They lie to get you in their arms. Eventually these kinds of liars will confess the truth when they feel safe in your love for him. This isn't exactly the same as the straight-up pathological liar. Your sweet little liar is lying to cover up his insecurities. He feels he doesn't measure up to your expectations so he lies and create them. But the sweet little liar will confess when confronted with his lies and maybe even tell you why he told them to begin with. He lied to get you in his life. Simple as that. Men have been doing this since time immemorial. He didn't set up the game he is forced to play anymore than you. The social power structure of the sexes is a cruel game but nonetheless it must be played in the search for a suitable mate. He isn't the kind to tell lies that could endanger your life or livelihood. He will even lie to spare your feelings. He truly wants you as to why he's lying.

I'm not saying it's right. I'm merely pointing out his reason for doing it. It's up to you to decide whether it's worth it to continue the relationship or keep dating him once you learn the truth. His fear of losing you is what prompt his lies. This type of liar doesn't lie about the important things like where he lives; what he does for a living and etc., because they are lying to get and keep you not to manipulate you or drive you away.

Chapter 47

__TALK TO YOUR MAN. TELL HIM HOW YOU FEEL. WHAT YOU WANTS. HE IS NOT A MIND READER.__

Since most of the readers of this book will likely be women. I want to tell you something that's very, very important. Tell men what you want. Don't expect them to know what you want. Even in bed, tell them. Open your mouth and talk and tell him what you want. Only a woman-hating cuck will find you as being out of your place as a woman. The very type of guy we are trying our very damnedest best to avoid. I realized this dilemma was created from centuries of women not being able to say what they wanted without being labeled negative. If you want to go to a certain place, then tell him. If you want a certain expensive or non-expensive item. Then tell him. If you want sex and is too shy to tell him. Develop little hints so he will know everytime you do that is when you want sex. A man who is attuned to you will soon learn what rubbing his chest a certain way means. Or your little smiles and glances means. Lovers can often communicate without speaking a word. Haven't you seen couples who have been married for years talk to each other without ever saying a word? But there are times you need to tell him what's on your mind. He can not read your mind.

Chapter 48

<u>ARE YOU WILLING TO BE THE ONE?</u>

A note to the men who may be reading this book if a woman you meet and her tone is very negative and dark towards men! Don't, whatever you do, just assumed it has something to do with her father. In most cases it has nothing at all to do with her father. The father thing is a mostly a lie and a myth and comes straight out of books and magazines that exploits women. It's a cheap cop out as many other things men say to avoid the responsibility of their actions. It has mostly to do with the men whom she met, believed and loved who took advantage of her heart. A heart can only be mistreated but for so long before it grows cold and callous. In most case, she stepped out into the dating world a warm, sweet, cheerful person with lots of love to give because that is *how* she saw her father treat her mother and assumed all guys were good guys like good old dad. That was her first fatal mistake. So, instead of making half-assed, chauvinist assumptions are *you* willing to show her that you aren't like the men she has been meeting. Yes, it's going to take work on the male's part too in order to find love. It's not going to just fall in your lap simply because you're a guy and society have told you all your life it would. You're old enough now to know it's all a lie. Those predeterminations were based upon the rules of a patriarch system that is slowly eroding away. Where women were forced into relationships. She probably has been burnt many times and learned to protect herself she by putting all men in the same box but if no man is brave enough to show her she's wrong. Then what's the point in pointing it out? Are you willing to be her Neo, her knight in the burnished armor? Show her that there are really loving, genuine, kind and respectful men out there! And she's looking at one. That the other guys in her life were just little boys and you are a man?

There are many women who have been raised by decent fathers and do not know how to look out for the wolves for they have never encountered them until out on their own. So yes, she got burnt a lot of times and maybe a lot reluctant to let anyone hurt her again. But are you man enough to be patience with her and show her what real love feels like? Or are you going to be like the men I described here who does nothing but bitch and complain about what she isn't? Love is made in the heart not in the bedroom. To find true love one must be willing to give true love. Are you man enough to help her heal?

There would be no real need for a book like this one had not men turned what nature intended to be easy, something as natural as breathing and eating into a damn weapon, a battlefield with all the lying, cheating, disrespect, dishonor, manipulations, hate and all sorts of negative emotions. Yes, the patriarch system can and does exploit women but it can not make them love men. This is where men have to stand up and say enough is enough. And try to understand what women goes through under this oppressive system.

THE MALE PRIVILEDGE CHECKLIST

To further advocate my point as to why women needs to break the shackles on our minds and hearts and start to put themselves first. I am quoting this well written article by Peggy McIntosh. The article was written nearly 20 years ago and much haven't changed since. If anything, things have become worse.

An Unabashed Imitation of an Article by Peggy McIntosh.

purpose, so long as the acknowledgment of Peggy McIntosh's work for inspiring this list is not removed25.)

In 1990, Wellesley College professor Peggy McIntosh wrote an essay called "White Privilege: Unpacking the Invisible Knapsack". McIntosh observes that whites in the U.S. are "taught to see racism only in individual acts of meanness, not in invisible systems conferring dominance on my group." To illustrate these invisible systems, McIntosh wrote a list of 26 invisible privileges whites benefit from.

As McIntosh points out, men also tend to be unaware of their own privileges as men. In the spirit of McIntosh's essay, I thought I'd compile a list similar to McIntosh's, focusing on the invisible privileges benefiting men.

Since I first compiled it, the list has been posted several times on Internet discussion groups. Very helpfully, many people have suggested additions to the checklist. More commonly, of course, critics (usually, but not always, male) have pointed out men have disadvantages too – being drafted into the army, being expected to suppress emotions, and so on. These are indeed bad things – but I never claimed that life for men is all ice cream sundaes. Pointing out that men are privileged in no way denies that sometimes bad things happen to men.

In the end, however, it is men and not women who make the most money; men and not women who dominate the government and the corporate boards; men and not women who dominate virtually all of the most powerful positions of society. And it is women and not men who suffer the most from intimate violence and rape; who are the most likely to be poor; who are, on the whole, given the short end of patriarchy's stick. As Marilyn Frye has argued, while men are harmed by patriarchy, women are oppressed by it.

Several critics have also argued that the list somehow victimizes women. I disagree; pointing out problems is not the same as perpetuating them. It is not a "victimizing" position to fight against injustice; we can't fight injustice if we refuse to acknowledge it exists.

An internet acquaintance of mine once wrote, "The first big privilege which whites, males, people in upper economic classes, the able bodied, the straight (I think one or two of those will cover most of us) can work to alleviate is the privilege to be oblivious to privilege." This checklist is, I hope, a step towards helping men to give up the "first big privilege."

The Male Privilege Checklist

1. My odds of being hired for a job, when

competing against female applicants, are probably skewed in my favour. The more prestigious the job, the larger the odds are skewed.

2. I can be confident that my co-workers won't think I got my job because of my sex —even though that might be true.

3. If I am never promoted, it's not because of my sex.

4. If I fail in my job or career, I can feel sure this won't be seen as a black mark against my entire sex's capabilities.

5. The odds of my encountering sexual harassment on the job are so low as to be negligible.

6. If I do the same task as a woman, and if the measurement is at all subjective, chances are people will think I did a better job.

7. If I'm a teen or adult, and if I can stay out of prison, my odds of being raped are so low as to be negligible.

8. I am not taught to fear walking alone after dark in average public spaces. If I have children but do not provide primary care for them, my

masculinity will not be called into question.

9. If I choose not to have children, my masculinity will not be called into question.

10. If I have children and provide primary care for them, I'll be praised for extraordinary parenting if I'm even marginally competent.

11. If I have children and pursue a career, no one will think bad of me If pursues my career instead of rearing the children and will think I'm selfish for not staying at home.

12. If I seek political office, my relationship with my children, or who I hire to take care of them, will probably not be scrutinized by the press.

13. Chances are my elected representatives are mostly people of my own sex. The more prestigious and powerful the elected position, the more likely this is to be true.

14. I can be somewhat sure that if I ask to see "the person in charge," I will face a person of my own sex. The higher-up in the organization the person is, the surer I can be.

15. As a child, chances are I was encouraged to be more active and outgoing than my sisters.

16. As a child, I could choose from an almost infinite variety of children' media featuring positive, active, non-stereotyped heroes of my own sex. I never had to look for it; male heroes were the default.

17. As a child, chances are I got more teacher attention than girls who raised their hands just as often.

18. If my day, week or year is going badly, I need not ask of each negative episode or situation whether or not it has sexist overtones.

19. I can turn on the television or glance at the front page of the newspaper and see people of my own sex widely represented, every day, without exception.

20. If I'm careless with my financial affairs it won't be attributed to my sex.

21. If I'm careless with my driving it won't be attributed to my sex.

22. I can speak in public to a large group without putting my sex on trial.

23. If I have sex with a lot of people, it won't make me an object of contempt or derision.

24. There are value-neutral clothing choices available to me; it is possible for me to choose clothing that doesn't send any particular message to the world.

25. My wardrobe and grooming are relatively cheap and consume little time.

26. If I buy a new car, chances are I'll be offered a better price than a woman buying the same car.

27. If I'm not conventionally attractive, the disadvantages are relatively small and easy to ignore.

28. I can be loud with no fear of being called a shrew. I can be aggressive with no fear of being called a bitch.

29. I can ask for legal protection from violence that happens mostly to men without being seen as a selfish special interest, since that kind of

violence is called "crime" and is a general social concern. (Violence that happens mostly to women is usually called "domestic violence" or "acquaintance rape," and is seen as a special interest issue.)

30. I can be confident that the ordinary language of day-to-day existence will always include my sex. "All men are created equal…," mailman, chairman, freshman, he.

31. My ability to make important decisions and my capability in general will never be questioned depending on what time of the month it is.

32. I will never be expected to change my name upon marriage or questioned if i don't change my name.

33. The decision to hire me will never be based on assumptions about whether or not I might choose to have a family sometime soon.

34. Every major religion in the world is led primarily by people of my own sex. Even God, in most major religions, is usually pictured as being male.

35. Most major religions argue that I should be

the head of my household, while my wife and children should be subservient to me.

36. If I have a wife or girlfriend, chances are we'll divide up household chores so that she does most of the labour, and in particular the most repetitive and unrewarding tasks.

37. If I have children with a wife or girlfriend, chances are she'll do most of the childrearing, and in particular the most dirty, repetitive and unrewarding parts of childrearing.

38. If I have children with a wife or girlfriend, and it turns out that one of us needs to make career sacrifices to raise the kids, chances are we'll both assume the career sacrificed should be hers.

39. Magazines, billboards, television, movies, pornography, and virtually all of media are filled with images of scantily clad women intended to appeal to me sexually. Such images of men exist, but are much rarer.

40. I am not expected to spend my entire life 20-40 pounds underweight.

41. If I am heterosexual, it's incredibly unlikely

that I'll ever be beaten up by a spouse or lover.

42. I have the privilege of being unaware of my male privilege.

That's an awful lot of privileges simply because you were born with a penis. For no other reason. Not that you are exceptional special in any other way. Not that you are bright, intelligent or even a good person. I do not buy it that the entire other half of the human race do not see anything seriously wrong with this seriously imbalance and wish they would quit bringing God into it. No one has ever proven if God is a male or female so why do we assume God is male?

But there's more. Another side to this coin that is so very rarely talked about that most people in America have paid very little attention to it. Because it only affects women of color.

In January 2017, there was a great feminist march on Washington D.C. but if anyone noted there wasn't many women of color there. Why not? Because the white feminist movement doesn't address their problems. It's mostly about "I'm so sick of my man's bullshit I could scream."

Guess what?! Everyone is so sick of the bullshit and have been screaming they are sick of it since 1492. But the only way to make a movement work is to bring all women into it and look squarely at what they are saying. They deals with racism and sexism in a way a white woman can not even begun to comprehend. No one is blaming you, the white woman for the oppressive system so it would serve you well if you stop behaving as if everyone is blaming you everytime it's mentioned. Stopping behaving also means stop agreeing with things you know are wrong but go along with it for whatever reason. Going along with it doesn't make things better for you. The original suffragists didn't bow out because their men didn't' like what they were doing. It makes them worse. Oppressors go after and eliminate everyone who may be an ally to you and when all the other groups of women have turned their backs on you then you have no allies. That's why it's vital to listen even if you don't fully understand what the woman of another ethnic group is saying. Your chances of ending up dead after a simple traffic stop is very slim. But with African American and many others, this is a very real agenda. It happens.

S

In a 1989 study by Dr. Peggy McIntosh, Ph.D, Associate Director of the Wellesley College Center for Research on Women, describes white privilege as "an invisible package of unearned assets, which I can count on cashing in each day, but about which I was 'meant' to remain oblivious. White privilege is like an invisible weightless knapsack of special provisions, maps, passports, code books, visas, clothes, tools, and blank checks"

The conclusions based on these educational studies is why I'm presenting to further prove my point as to why especially women of color need to learn to use sex as a weapon. Some are so obsessed with getting a man that you will do anything to get him without the slightly clue as to why you are doing these ridiculous things. Failing to realize it's mental and social conditioning that goes all the way back to the feudal system that strive until World War I and with women of African descent much of it goes back to slavery and beyond.

Another major reason I mentioned these facts is that it sadden me to hear and often read the very hateful and disgusting comments made by women to other women. ALL women (just because they are women) share a common experiences in life that erode their self-esteem as human beings. The glass ceiling of equal opportunity has still not been broken. Ladies, let's unite and support those like each other who do their very best to help all of us! Stop the bickering, crazy cat fights, petty insults and criticisms (possibly motivated by jealousy?). It achieves nothing but what who those invented it intended that it achieves.

Chapter 49

WOMEN OF COLOR

I created a chapter especially women of color because I've so often seen well educated beautiful black women with someone she really needs to kick to the curb. If I can see it from mere observation, I'm certain she already knows that. Why are you with someone who is not pulling you upward? You already have a list of over two hundred points to deal with from the moment you are born. You've more crazy shit to deal with than any other woman in America. So why are you with someone who doesn't respect you and is merely adding to the list of shit to deal with? Won't help you better yourself. Won't try to better himself. Don't hand me the excuse about discrimination in America. It's very real and I do not deny it exist. But if he truly applied himself he can go further than you for all having a penis and nothing more. You face racism and sexism and succeed. He doesn't face sexism. You are still at the very lowest rank of the social economic ladder. Foreigners from another country and come here and do better than you who has roots here since 1619.

Black women desperately needs to adapt the same attitude as everyone else. "Forget you." By their actions, that's exactly what everyone else is saying to you. Including the black man. If that wasn't the case... why the moment he gets a million coins to jingles in his pocket he heads straight out of your arms into the arms of a white woman or any woman but a black woman? If if was love as some often cries. They would've found each other before he became famous. No, it's the power of sex at work and she happens to know how to wield it.

Even so-called black music and networks degrades black women. When in popular black movies always present a fair skinned black woman as the love interest? Why is that? I see it this way. To dark skinned black girls that's clearly saying *nobody want you*. It's ok to have sex with you or even father children by you but you aren't pretty or white enough to marry.

One the dumbest things I've ever seen is so many young black women defending entertainers who put them down. How are lyrics rapping, "beat that bitch down or smack that whore," an euthenics expression of one's culture when the video accompanying it has black women dancing and twerking far more promiscuous than many professional strippers? It doesn't matter who is doing the exploiting, it's still wrong. One form doesn't justify another.

Some may ask what has all this to do with getting a man and holding on to him? Everything. Absolutely everything. The reason being is that in America one isn't viewed as beautiful unless she is white or a lighter race than those of African descendants. Honestly, if we all would admit the truth. We all know that is hogwash. Black women are the most beautiful women in the world. But after centuries of cucks telling them they are nothing and years of constantly being told you aren't beautiful has damaged many women of darker races opinion of themselves is why we see so many with men who are not good for them. As to why she accepts behavior from men that's destructive to her life. She doesn't see herself as beautiful mainly because of steady stream of being abused and mistreated. It has gone on for so long that she sees herself as her oppressors say she is.

This image is everywhere. The media blares it in her face all day every fucking day as it is their god given right to do it. If an ethnic woman is portrayed in a movie, book, music video, or etc. It's almost, always a stereotypical role. The only movies that does well in the box office are those where she's portrayed in negative stereotypical projections. So little wonder she may have a self-image problem.

She can't arrange to be in the company of people of her race most of the time if she moves up in the world. She has to go out and find them.

She can't go shopping alone most of the time, pretty well assured that she won't be followed or harassed.

She can't turn on the television, sign online or open to

the front page of the newspaper or magazine, book and see people of her race widely represented.

When she's told about her national heritage or about "civilization," She's told that other people made it what it is. It completely leaves out the fact that genocide and slavery made it what it is. It completely leaves out she is a descendant of people who were kidnapped and forced into labor and usually dead by age 30. Is what made it what it is.

She can't be sure that when her children are given curricular materials that these studies will testify to the existence of her race.

She can't go into a music store or video game store and count on finding the music of her race represented, or video games where the women of race aren't readily portrayed as easy and promiscuous. She can't into a supermarket and readily find the food she grew up with, she can't walk into any old beauty shop and find some one who can deal with her hair. With African American women, the natural state of their hair is taught it is something to be ashamed of. Ridiculed and have even known to cost many of them their jobs. During slavery, she had to keep it cover or faced a lashing.

She can't use checks, credit cards, or cash, and not be subtly questioned if she stole them. She must show everything short of a DNA test result to prove she is who she says she is and to provide proof that they are indeed hers'. Or worse the clerk hopes the card or check is declined so he or she can snobbishly tell her it is no good. She can't count on her skin color <u>not</u> working against her in the agenda of financial responsibility. No one else is single handed blamed for the national deficit but yet receive less of the slice of the pie. The social economic programs created by President Roosevelt were designed to assistance the poor whites not women of color and no one came out against it back then; it didn't become a political battle cry until the programs begin to assistance women of color.

Some of the very same politicians decrying these programs, were aided by them in their youth. These programs are what landed them where they sat today. But never mind all that. Too many women of color are using them today to improve their lot in life therefore there must a strict astringent placed on them to be sure they aren't cheating to get them.

She is constantly made acutely aware that her body shape, her natural body movement, her presentation in public, or even her natural body odor is a reflection on her race.

She is told her concerns about racism are selfish, self-interested or self-seeking. She needs to get over it or go back to where she came from. Never mind not being conscious of it existence can end her life. If she is killed in a derogatory form, then it's her sex life not the probe for her killer you hear about.

She can't take a job or enroll in a college without

knowing an affirmative action policy is the only reason she's there.

She can't be late to a meeting without having the lateness reflect on her race. After dealing with 400 years of bullshit. It's a miracle she showed up at all.

She can't choose any public accommodation with out fearing that people of her race cannot get in or will be mistreated. Or she maybe the only person of her race there.

She always asked to speak for all of the people of her racial group. As if she supposed to know every single person in her race and what they think and do.

She can never be pretty sure that if having a problem and ask to talk with the "person in charge" She will be facing a person of her race. In most cases she won't. Most of the time the person in charge doesn't take her complaint seriously because of her race or deliberately deny addressing the issue especially if it is beneficial to her. Sure, it will be addressed very quickly if the sordid outcome is going to be malignant to her. Usually the person in charge, then can't attend it fast enough. So why is that? If racism and sexism isn't the culprit?

If a traffic cop pulls her over, she has every right to be afraid even if the cop is of her own race. Polices aren't immune to the same social mental conditioning any more than anyone else. Or if the IRS audits her tax return, which in most cases aren't worth the bother. She can't be sure she haven't been singled out because of her race. Again, these employees came from the same society which has systemically victimized her for years. They aren't going to put on a different set of morals the moment they enter that building and dispose of them when they leave.

When buying for her loved ones she can't easily buy posters, postcards, picture books, greeting cards, dolls, toys, and children' magazines featuring people of her race. I've picked and read many books where the main characters are nonwhite but the book cover shows a white person. And the catch to this if a woman of color she wants to do well in the literary world then she must write about stereotypical characters. If she expects to be perceived well. She must write about race and nothing else. If she writes about romantic relationships it must be about her female characters going nuts over a black or white guy who is treating her like shit. Or even her own race will not buy and read her work. To me, that's pretty much saying that she isn't allowed to think and dream about anything else. So, why is that?

She can't go the drug store for a minor cut and choose blemish cover or bandages in "flesh" color and have them more or less match her skin hue. Even make up companies are way behind in this agenda. Very few make cosmetic becoming women of color

She can't do well in a challenging situation without being called a credit to her race. But if she does poorly it will definitely be accredited to her race. Simply viewed as she was expected to fail because of her race.

She can't openly do and say ethnic things without making others uncomfortable.

If her family has moved up in the world, she can't walk into a classroom and know she will not be the only member of her race there. In many cases this is the neighborhood's first close up encounter with a person of color. So that lone child is representing her entire race to these people and yet expected to do the same work and excel in an environment that merely tolerates her. She must work four times as hard as everyone else for the same education which will some day provide a job where she will make four times less than everyone else but yet is still expected to make ends meet.

If she's accepted at an Ivy League school, she can't enroll in a class at college and safely assume that the majority of her professors will be of her race. On many campuses, there's isn't a single member of the faculty of her own race within yelling distance.

So, the next time you see a frustrated woman of color cussing someone out good and righteous please bear in mind it isn't just an African American thing, an Asian thing, a Mexican thing, or a Native American thing. It's a women of color thing. She is tired of being shitted on by everyone and everyone has a breaking point. These are all the things she deals with in her life from cradle to the grave which are erupting out of her mouth at the moment. So, stop and put yourself in her shoes. How would you react if you had to deal with this mega load of stupid bullshit every day? Wouldn't you be cussing everyone out too who pissed you off? It's very easy to sat on your behind and say what you wouldn't do, say, or how you wouldn't act when you don't have to deal with it.

"What has all this to do with learning to wield the power of sex?" Some of you are asking by now? Every thing. In order to wield power you have to know the structure of it and how it works and who it works against. If you don't want to take the time to learn these things then you will be in the dark when you are confronted with one of the various forms of them. Like it or not racist spill over into the dating world and shape and forms how people think, feels and react in certain situations.

All of the reasons listed above is why I strongly advise women of color not to become involved in the sex market. It's far too dangerous and you have no protection. You can not change anyone's perception of you. It's too ingrained. But you can work to protect yourself by not becoming involved in it. The quick money isn't worth your life.

No, I don't advise against interracial dating. It's great for real love knows no color or gender. I said dating, not stripping. I have something against women of color getting involved in the sex market because they have no protection. But please be aware when starting to interracial date there are some racists out there who will date women of color and a few have even married women of color but still... deep down inside he has never really changed his view of the her race. And don't be surprised when it comes out for it is bind to eventually come out.

I know all of this is a lot for anyone to digest and live with. But African American women live with it every day and have been doing so since 1619. For those who believed the talking cucks that she isn't beautiful and desirable she needs to work on building her self-esteem and looking beyond her community for love. Despite with everything said about her and done to her she has still managed to rise to the top. It takes one helluva woman to do that. So ignore the cucks, the media and the naysayers who says no one want you. They're lying big time. It's nothing more than the same old brain-washing that was tried centuries ago. It's merely wearing a new suit. Other men who aren't obsessed with being a racist bastard finds you very beautiful. So there's no need for you to still be beholding to a system that was never designed to aid you.

Make the black man practice what he preaches. From what I see it's all lip service with no sustenance to back it up. If he REALLY wants to be with you make him do better or stop sleeping with him if he won't do better.

Considering the history of African Americans in America. I know where your clutch in holding him up is coming from. But far too many are exploiting the black woman's justified fear for his life and well-being while not giving a rat's ass how she feels. If someone doesn't give a rat's ass how you feel, then return the benignity. Stop being everyone's shoulder to cry on. Take care of yourself first and then if you have any time and energy left is when you allow others into your life. Anyone who doesn't value your presence isn't worthy of it.

Chapter 50

STOP WASTING YOUR SWEET PRECIOUS TIME

Time is valuable and precious. We all have an expiration date and none of us know when. We aren't stamped like a carton of milk or loaf of bread as to when we will expire. So make the best of every hour as if it's your last. Stop wasting time on people who aren't worth one of your hours or minutes.

Stop trying to figure out the guy who shuts you out when he's in a shitty ass mood. What did you do to cause his behavior? That's none of your concern. He's an asshole. Shit comes out of assholes so he's acting like what he is. Stop worrying about whether it has anything to do with you. The guy that will walk past you like you're an apparition or replies one-word answers, like you're nothing to him, even though he acted like you were everything yesterday when his day was going well. He's a cuck. This is a form of manipulation. He wants to pursue him. Most people who behave such as this are actually a narcissist.

Stop wasting time with the guy who had a nasty ex-girlfriend or wife but takes her behavior out on you, eventhus, you aren't anything like her. It's not your fault he refused to leave her abusive ass. This type of guy will play the victim and acts like he's damaged, and repays your kindness with wrath. Get out! He has too much baggage from his last relationship. He's not ready to let anyone else inside. Be more than just a warm body in a bed.

Stop wasting time with the guy that makes you wonder if your phone is malfunctioning or did you pay your phone bill, because you haven't gotten a text back from him yet, even though you messaged him two hours to two days ago and you can see that he's been active on Facebook or Twitter over the last twenty minutes. He's isn't worth a second thought. Move on. Find someone new.

Stop wasting time with the guy that gets you excited about spending time with him, and then tells you that he's so sorry but he forgot that you two made plans, or that something unexpectedly came up and he has to cancel. And he does it...Every. Damn. Time. Again, never stick around for it to happen twice. Find something to do other than sit around and wait for him.

His actions are telling you, you are a very low priority on his list.

Stop wasting time with the guy that only gives you bits and pieces of his life story, even though you've opened up to him about everything from your family secrets to your childhood pets, everything from your darkest fears to your brightest passions. Which you shouldn't have done. Learn to keep your mouth shut. He hiding something big time or could be just not truly interested in you or find you boring but this is better than being completely alone. People don't leave in the spur of a moment. It has long been fathoming in their minds and when they finds the one they wish to be with, they leave.

Stop wasting time with the guy that can't keep his narrations straight. The guy who you know is lying because he gives you different 'concepts' each time you talk to him and then swears that you're remembering things wrongly. He tries to convince you that you're the crazy one. No, he's not crazy. He thinks he's clever. Lies are hard to keep track of. Much harder than the truth.

He's simply a manipulative bastard. Get away from him. This is how he operates. Who know? He might try to "Gaslight" you.

Stop wasting time with the guy who calls you two, three, four times when *he* wants to see you and won't take no for an answer and then does a complete 360 degree turn around when you initiate contact by ignoring every one of your texts. He ignores you because he only cares about what he wants in the moment. Usually he is already in a relationship or married and the urgency and persistence is that he have to see you before she returns.

Stop wasting time with the guy who only wants to talks to you through Skype, Snapchat or other instant messages, because he isn't interested in having nor does he plan on developing a meaningful conversation, let alone a relationship with you — he only wants to get a glance at the outfit that you're wearing and to test the waters to see if you'll send nudes images or any at all. Some collect these images. It's a hobby.

Stop wasting time with the guy who only posts party photos of himself with a drink in his hand. He brags about how much he can chug without passing out. He will only contacts you when he's drunk. He thinks being inebriated deserves a medal of honor. Drunks do not make good partners. You aren't AA, you can't change him.

Stop wasting time with a man that acts as if you committed a cardinal sin if you mention another guy, eventhus he have many selfies with his arms around women and interrupts your conversation to check his beeping phone that you know has girls on the other line. This is so juvenile. Granting, it's very infantile, it's still a manipulation tactic used to control and condition you to accept his behavior.

Stop wasting time with a guy who is always checking himself out. Who looks into the mirror to check his appearance more than he looks at you, because he's more concerned with the way the world views him than the way that you view him. He knows he's hot and relies on his looks to get him through life. Get out after the first date for he is going to render your self-esteem to shreds. The relationships must always be all about him.

Stop wasting time with the guy whose moods plainly says he doesn't care whether you stay in his life or not. The guy who keep you up all when you should be getting beauty sleep, replaying in your mind what's his guff? You replay the scene over and over trying to figure out whether he likes you or not — whether he cares or not. Stop it. He plainly told you by his actions how he feels. **Stop it** and go the fuck to sleep because you deserves so much more than that guy.

Chapter 51

DON'T EXCUSE, ROMANTICIZE, NOR GLORIFY ABUSE AND UNHEALTHY, TOXIC BEHAVIORS.

It's impossible to talk about wielding sexual power,

dating and relationships without mentioning this subject. Some of the most popular movies and books out today glorify and romanticize abuse and toxic behavior. Especially sexual abuse. It has gone as far as making it the norm. It has been made into an acceptable normal. As if it is an acceptable part of a relationship. It's not. It's as dysfunctional as a relationship can get.

It troubles me that so many women totally accept and put up with abusive toxic partners as a sign he loves them. They accept the belittling, the ultimatums, the manipulations, the slaps, the blows. Even some of the strongest, most accomplished women accepts this sort of put down and abuse. Why? When she has her own everything. So why is she accepting the abusive? The reality is this toxic behavior is made into a normal part of relationships and even viewed as romantic. That it supposedly speaks volumes in how much he loves you. Well, if it does I don't want anyone to love me so much he must slap my face, scream at me until my ears bleed, or belittle me. He can keep that kind of love. I can do without it.

And to make matters worst these women claim the world that they deserved it! When you accept abuse you aren't wielding power. You are giving up power. The abuse is not about love. It's all about power and control.

I realized that we are flooded with occurrences of venomous relationships from the media and the pop culture. So much of this crap flow in inundations that it eventually numbs us to the fact it is actually abuse. There are people who get into relationships who really do conduct these behaviors. It supposedly shows much power they can wield and how hot they must be for anyone to willing accept it just be with them. There's so much manipulations that it has become normalized. The deprecating is done repetitive so often that the person start to believe that this is their true worth. That's the sole purpose of degrading someone; to destroy or tear down their self-worth so they will accept your bullshit. It has nothing to do with love. No one who love you makes you cry. Someone who loves dry your tears. Not become the source of them.

Once I was listening to a hit song by a popular artist who was singing about her man lying to her and she knew he was lying but it was ok because she liked the pain his lies were causing her. I was thinking, *"Girl, you seriously need your head examined by a psychiatrist to learn why you like for someone to hurt you."* I saw this the abuse was being used as a mask of a much deeper problem, that could potentially turn deadly. It's an illusion of love was being overshadowed by a pretense and tumultuous, addictive romance. Real romance isn't a tumorous whirlwind of pain.

For those trapped in the gamut of negativity, get out. It doesn't get better. Many have been in it so long she believe she deserves the pain, and that she is supposed to accept it. She starts to lose herself to abuse.

The romantic pleads and promises in the nephrotoxic relationship often keeps the woman from leaving: "**I promise, I swear I love you so much you makes me**

crazy." Is an ever popular one. No, the person was already crazy when you met him. You gullibly ignored the warning signs believing your love could change him.

"I'll never hit you again." Hit once, they will hit again and again. Verbal abuse usually starts before the slaps and punches. The disrespect, lies, belittling and insults are all paving the way for the fist.

"I'd never do nothing to hurt him. He didn't mean it. He was just upset. I need to learn to not talk back when he's angry." This is usually the response of a woman whom anyone is trying to tell she need to get the hell out of there. Usually by now the couple are in each other's face expectorating venom when they speak to each other. Her replies are usually along the line of: "He loves me. He doesn't mean it when he say those horrible things. He doesn't mean it when his actions got out of hand." Yes, he did or he wouldn't have said them or done. All these answer goes back to low self-esteem.

I have pondered over the belief, there will be better days if she tough it. That this is nothing more than a storm she must weather through. I know the belief of toughening up to a horrible marriage or relationship out comes from women' low status in life. But that was then. And this is now. Those women had no choice. We do, they fought, marched, protested and some died to give us a choice which we are throwing unappreciative back in their dead faces.

There's a certain amount of codependency in all relationships, but the amount remains healthy. There are couple who are addiction to each other but there's no violence in the relationship. They simply can't keep their hands off each other. (in a loving way) But when codependency, violence, control, and manipulation are deemed to be romantic. A sign of love, then this is when the woman could question herself and ask herself why does she view negativity as love?

S

Money, great looks and even stellar accomplishments

doesn't always equate self-esteem and knowing your self worth. I know society says it does but it doesn't. If that were true women with all these things would not end up or remain in abusive relationships. We as a society has been brainwashed to believe that accomplishment equals self worth. When the two doesn't always mean the same thing. We has been brainwashed to believe that low esteem equates being poor or a low achievers in the manners in which society defines a high achiever. But many so-called low achievers are actually very happy people and have a healthy self esteem.

I am fully aware that the meaning of this acceptance is a way of supposedly saying that the endurance of such treatment is solid proof of a love so powerful it can weather through all the challenges and shortcomings of loving someone. The only thing it proves is that the abuser has some serious issues and you need to get away from him. So stop romanticizing abuse and unhealthy behaviors. They aren't romantic, they aren't love and nor are they are test of the strength of love. They are toxic and dysfunctional. Nothing more.

I'm a firm believer of when people show you their true self, believe them. For as much as you do not wish to believe them. Believe them for they know themselves far better than you.

Chapter 52

MEN WHO WATCH PORN ARE TERRIBLE LOVERS AND PARTNERS.

It has been proven again and again that men who watch porn are terrible lovers. Simple as that! Porn isn't about mastering the art of becoming a good lover. It's about instantly satisfying a primitive urge just as prostitution.

Prior to the internet, finding and using pornography required patience, even a bit of imagination and getting up going into a store to actually buy it. There were no such thing as free downloads. The closest thing most boys found to porn was mail order catalogue of underwear models from mail order companies like Macy's' or Victoria Secret, whose catalogs infrequently came in the mail. He had to use his mind and make his imagination work harder at unlocking the delightful image beneath the underwear. But a new catalog once every few weeks was far too intermittent for most males. However after the arrival of internet porn those days of waiting for porn and teasing their imagination are gone.

At this very moment, I can safely bet at this moment 10 out a hundred men in Western Civilization and beyond—have his hands on an electronic device loaded with an unreal but lusty pornographic material ready to arouse his lust and blow his loins wide open. Never stopping to think how it influence his attitude toward real women. I have learned that's what some of all the snarky attitudes online toward women are all about. So how is a real woman to compete with that? You can't. So even don't try. It's not worth the effort. But I am writing on this subject because people need to know how it effects reality.

These statistics are disturbing:

• Every second, 28,258 Internet users are viewing

pornography.

• American children begin viewing pornography at an average age of 10-11.

• The pornography industry is a $97 billion industry worldwide.

• Men are 543% more likely to look at porn than are women.

• More than 1 in 5 searches on mobile devices are for pornography.

Porn is ubiquitous and very lucrative business. You might be surprised who uses online porn. There are men who've spent countless hours over many years caught in the sticky pornographic web. You would never imagine who maybe using it.

For some men a great sexual encounters with a woman is a rare luxury. But heir computer or IPhone, on the other hand, is all too willing to dance for them, undress for them, tease them, fictional lick, suck, screw them with all the indulge being on them, whatever they want it, any time they want. They don't have to be concern with anyone's feelings but their own. That's the problem as to why their encounters are rare. Lack of empathy and feelings. Women has an inherent ability to sense when a male has no feelings. Why most won't use it is? Been taught for so long not to use it. That's his feelings are more important than her own.

S

Most users do not, in general think they have an addiction. Just as most drug users or alcoholics doesn't think they have one either but yet porn viewers spend days and weeks using internet pornography every night to quickly arouse and then satiate themselves. There and then just to fall asleep. Again, there's no woman to ask anything or do pillow talk.

According to study, most watch it up to an hour or more in bed before becoming exhausted enough to fall asleep. This study was conducted by recording the length of time a viewer stays on the sites

There's nothing wrong with masturbation but when it starts to take the place of a relationship with a real live human. It's time to stop it. Most do not realize that modern pornography can become a serious detriment to everyone.

Here are vital reasons why men who are addictive to it need helps and could give up concordant use of pornography as a sexual stimulation:

Porn ruins men erections with actual women. Men, are unlike women who can keep going after one orgasm after another. With most men once they ejaculate, the act is over. He doesn't see her as being a human but an object as the images in his device and will response accordingly.

After using porn even moderately on a regular basis he

become unable to sustain erections with women as he once was. He's aroused as ever, but without the constantly changing visual erotic stimulation that porn provides, one woman's body won't hold his erotic focus. Real life sex becomes under stimulating.

Biologically, porn tunes men bodies to premature ejaculation. It turns him into a minute man which is someone no woman wants in her bed. Secretly, that is the culprit in many disastrous love making attempts where the magazines are telling her she need to do oh so many things to make herself desirable. No she doesn't. He simply needs to stop watching porn.

It attunes a man's body to quickly rise and climax. Where as with a real woman. Her aroused body doesn't stop moving so fast as a masturbating hand. And trying to bring her down from a sexual high is like trying to stop a tidal at full surge and men can't handle her sweltering moments and some will get angry and start to label her names all because of his own short comings.

After quitting porn, a man body's nervous system to

return to its natural state, a less hurried sexual pace and rhythm which he will enjoy whether he knows it or not much better than the drill hammer approach. A good lover know sex is much better unhurried.

Porn is nothing but a prop. It's a sorry ass excuse from interacting powerfully with actual women. Our own patriarchal society and those worldwide has never taught men how to relate to and interact with women as a human being without taking her sexuality into the concept. Most men, in generally do not know how to interact powerfully with women and surely not as a mature healthy man. They fail to step up to women they're attracted to in effective and honorable, respectful ways. So many let their secret crushes slip away forever into the dark painful cave of anguish. They need to grow up and learn that is part of life. Nearly everyone has had a crush on someone they never let it saw the light of day. But we don't dive head first into perversion because of it.

The other day I watched several men walked right pass a very attractive woman carrying an arm load of parcels. One was walking parallel with her and didn't as so much turn his head and offer her a hand. This really had nothing to do with gender...it had a lot to do with common human decency.

I recently read in a magazine that masturbation can take the edge off all the frustration of dealing with real women. I'm still puzzled as to how this helps in dealing respectfully with women? How it helps in interactions with actual women? Are you going to masturbate everytime you are confronted by a woman? If that's the case...is it safe to shake your hand? This is bologna. This falls under the category of 'if advice makes no sense don't use it'. Men are taught this peculiar behavior they aren't born with it. Young boys interact with women as wholesome as they do men. Boys who are around well-adjusted men continues this normal interaction on into adulthood.

Porn is a fantasy world and if a male engage in it too soon, before his mind is mature enough to distinguish fictional from reality it creates unrealistic expectations of women. It has been proven it can be a major source of misogynistic and antagonistic attitudes toward women and girls.

Just from writing to men online I have found that porn make men think women should be easier to get into bed. It make think he will get laid more if he's more bold or clever, insulting, rude, making lewd compliments or more aggressive. This may work for some women but a woman with a healthy self-esteem this is a total turn off. Boldness with women is fine but still be a gentleman. Porn doesn't teach that. The activities only message is that women are here for one purpose and that is men pleasure.

Boldness is great but it could never be exercised to the point cost of alternating a man's genuine care and respect for women.

Another common scene that makes it difficult to make men understand that women in the real world doesn't behave as the women in porn is that the script is written for total male dominance. The women in porn let a man (or men) aggressively open them up and do whatever they want. They take close up shots of their mouths, vaginas or rectums, or with the woman on her knees beneath a penis in her mouth and according to the facial expression in video she is in sexual euphoria and happy and willing to be conquered and owned by a man, and do not mind displaying her body for all the world to see.

One of the most common scenes in porn and even in romance movies, novel and etc is that women response sexual to aggression. In my experience, actual women don't respond to male aggression by opening her legs. They only do that in fantasy world. And even if they do it in reality and sometimes they do – that doesn't create a bona fide loving relationship. It's usually out of fear not love. She's trying to appease him so he will not harm her. There's nothing romantic or loving about it.

I agree, we women are lusty, beautiful, sexy humans. We have a sexuality aspect the same as like men. But men need to taught how to relate us in deeper manner, ways that aren't always sexuality. The divine, wondrous feminine mystique of a woman that all men desperately crave to experience, is only available to men who have learn how to appreciate, love, and cherish a woman in her fullness of being a woman and that certainly doesn't happen in porn.

When men watch porn they supports oppressing one half of the human population. There's no other way to put it. They supports child abuse, human trafficking, sex slavery, rape, spousal and relationship abuse and in many case, the blackmailing of women. This happens to women all over the world not just in poor nations or poor neighborhoods.

Some may say my taste is tamed or soft porn but have not you still unwittingly saw videos on the average free porn site that were disturbing? Do you truly think a sane, free woman conducted that act? No, she didn't most likely it was forced.

Porn is abusive to women. In many scenes the men manipulate and even outright blackmail the women into unwanted forced sex in counterfeit cabs, bogus police officers handcuffing a woman to a bed or pipe. Phony doctors demands she strip in his office. The scenarios are endless with all having one thing in common. Female submission. Ironically, most people don't find it peculiar that the camera never shows the man's face; always the woman's. It's no great mystery why this is gone. The oppressor is always to remain faceless, random, annoymous. It's a symbolical representation of male domainate society.

There are countless criminal cases worldwide where people, mostly men, have been arrested and prosecuted for creating pornography with women they trafficked from other countries; women who were enslaved in buildings they can't leave; women kept in place by physical violence and threats of death and some are killed if she resist. Some are drugged and videoed and then threatened with exposure to their families and friends. Sadly most of these women keep quiet because we still live in a misogynistic society that isn't going to help her but berate or even harm her. So think of this everytime you watch porn. Whether you are watching videos where women are performing sex acts they were forced to do. If you knew would your tastes in porn be tamed. Truthfully but sadly, in most men it would not. I'm not male bashing. I'm simply speaking the truth.

It has been proven there's a direct link between porn and sexual crimes.

Don't let the temptation to watch porn cheat you out of a loving relationship. Those men are actors on a set. No real woman is going to do most of those things. Resist it.

There are couple whose relationships and marriages have ended because the man became un able to relate to a live woman so clearly nothing good ever comes from of the habit.

Men, have got to stop using porn as a quick fix. I know But it's also a cheap fix that deprive men of the basic of human nature. Love and fellowship with other humans. No amount of porn or fantasy can take the place of being in a relationship with someone who loves you. I know some couples even use it to spice up an otherwise dull sex life.

I read in a magazine where they listed many way to arouse your man. Sorry to say, but this is what's wrong with so many young men who don't have a physical problem as to why it takes so much to arouse him. A normal porn free, drug free man doesn't need anything to arouse him. All he needs is the woman to say 'yes'.

Find other ways to spice up your love life. Be

creative. Be romantic. Porn is easy as clicking a mouse. It's beneath our intelligence. It's not just hurting men; it's also hurting women.

Chapter 53

DECIDES WHAT YOU WANT AND GO AFTER IT.

The lesson of this is book is that there's always going to some one who disagree with you, criticize you, label you as long as you live. But do not let others' opinions stand in the way of your happiness. This book was written from research, life and mere observation of human being interacting with each other.

Reference

An Unabashed Imitation of an Article by Peggy McIntosh.